It is often assumed by those studying animal behaviour that the social system adopted by a species is a fixed product of natural selection. There is now an interesting body of evidence that this is not always the case, and that alternative forms of social organization may be adopted according to circumstance. In this book Professor Lott presents a contemporary overview of our current understanding of this phenomenon, and its implications for animal conservation and management. Those interested in social systems and more generally in animal behaviour and ecology, will find this book to be an invaluable source of information and ideas.

Cambridge Studies in Behavioural Biology

Intraspecific variation in the social
systems of wild vertebrates

Intraspecific Variation in the Social Systems of Wild Vertebrates

DALE F. LOTT

Department of Wildlife and Fisheries Biology
University of California
Davis, California 95616
USA

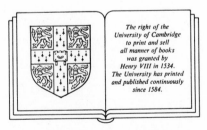

The right of the
University of Cambridge
to print and sell
all manner of books
was granted by
Henry VIII in 1534.
The University has printed
and published continuously
since 1584.

CAMBRIDGE UNIVERSITY PRESS

Cambridge

New York   Port Chester   Melbourne   Sydney

Published by the Press Syndicate of the University of Cambridge
The Pitt Building, Trumpington Street, Cambridge CB2 1RP
40 West 20th Street, New York NY 10011, USA
10 Stamford Road, Oakleigh, Melbourne 3166, Australia

First published 1991

Printed in Great Britain at the University Press, Cambridge

British Library cataloguing in publication data
Lott, Dale F.
Intraspecific variation in the social systems of wild
vertebrates.
1. Vertebrates. Intraspecific variation
I. Title   II. Series
596

Library of Congress cataloguing in publication data available
Lott, Dale F.
Intraspecific variation in the social systems of wild vertebrates
by Dale F. Lott.
    p.   cm. — (Cambridge studies in behavioural biology)
Includes bibliographical references and index.
ISBN 0-521-37024-8 (hardback)
1. Social behavior in animals.   2. Animal populations.
3. Vertebrates—Behavior.   4. Vertebrates—Variation.   I. Title.
II. Series.
QL775.L696   1990
596'.051—dc20   89-41345 CIP

ISBN 0 521 37024 8 hardback

PN

CONTENTS

PREFACE

Unexpected behavioral variation is noise. If it persists despite careful efforts to eliminate it, it becomes signal. Signal is described and analyzed, and its messages are decoded.

Intraspecific variation in social systems has recently become signal. Observations of different populations, or the same population at different times, increasingly revealed that social plasticity was common. Moreover, social system variation often appeared to be systematically and adaptively related to differences in ecological or demographic circumstances. The reports appear in a wide range of sources under a wide range of titles. This has limited the visibility and impact of intraspecific variation in social systems. But this variation creates opportunities for exciting and useful research to identify the environmental determinants and to analyze the proximate mechanisms that lead to social system variation. My efforts to aggregate this literature, and develop an overview and perspective on it prior to beginning a research program, started me down the road to this book.

It is exhilarating to begin a book about a rapidly expanding literature that appears in a variety of unexpected places. Finishing such a book is a bit depressing. The literature's degree of dispersal and rate of expansion ensure that important facts and ideas have escaped my notice or understanding. I encourage readers to call omissions to my attention.

ACKNOWLEDGEMENT

I was and remain astonished by the generosity so many people displayed in giving me so much help with this book. Several read the entire text of one or more versions. They include my academic editors Patrick Bateson and George Barlow, my Cambridge Press editors Alan Crowden and Sara Trevitt, my colleagues Benjamin Hart, Lynette Hart and Steven Minta, and the students who used an early draft as the text in a course: Christina Maher, Scott McWilliams, Michael Mooring, Elizabeth Jacobs, Deborah Jaques, Patrick Leonard, Ronald Swaisgood and Steven Towers. The following colleagues read and commented on individual chapters: Richard Coss, William Mason, Sally Mendoza, Robert Murphey, Donald Owings, and Peter Rodman. The manuscript and its author profited from discussions with Timothy Clutton-Brock, Nicholas Davies and Nicholas Macintosh. Christine Maher gave invaluable help with word processing and bibliography management and compiled the first draft of table one. Greg Kessler assisted in the literature search and bibliography. Katharine Marr drew the figures.

Special thanks to Laura for her support, encouragement and patience throughout the writing.

1

Introduction

Not so long ago it seemed that a species' social systems were fixed attributes. Each species was either territorial or not, was monogamous or polygynous or polyandrous, solitary or gregarious. Now we know that is not so. Golden-winged sunbirds (*Nectarinia reichenowi*) sometimes defend foraging territories, and at other times abandon those territories and forage in scramble competition organized by dominance relationships (Gill & Wolf, 1975). Dunnocks (*Prunella modularis*) breed monogamously, polyandrously, polygynously and polygynandrously (Davies & Lundberg, 1984). Some of their nestlings are fed by two adults, others by three (Davies & Houston, 1986).

These are not rare exceptions to an otherwise reliable rule. Several hundred examples of such intraspecific variation in vertebrate social systems are aggregated and summarized in chapters 2 and 3. Variation in social systems raises a number of questions: are these alternative strategies adaptive? What proximate mechanisms produce shifts from one system to another? Are some species more predisposed to social system variation than others? Does intraspecific variation in social systems provide a more rigorous test of socioecological hypotheses than differences between species? Can social plasticity help solve management and conservation problems? Will it create some? This book addresses these questions.

1.1   PLAN OF THE BOOK

This book has several goals. The first is to aggregate and summarize existing reports of intraspecific variation in the social systems of wild vertebrates. The second is to conduct a preliminary examination of

1

ultimate and proximate factors that might be acting as determinants of these variations. The third is to discuss the implications of social system variation for the way we analyze social systems. The fourth goal is to illuminate both the potential and the pitfalls of research on intraspecific variation in social systems.

1.2   HISTORY OF INTRASPECIFIC VARIATION IN SOCIAL SYSTEMS

Intraspecific variation in social systems is now an accepted part of our picture of animal social behavior. This was not always the case. For some time, the study of social behavior operated on the premise that social systems were a fixed feature of each species. Thus, species were said to be territorial or monogamous *per se*, rather than being described as territorial or monogamous in a certain place at a certain time. Deviations from these patterns were usually treated as aberrant. Some such variations have been treated as aberrant behavior which fortuitously revealed the function of the 'true' social systems. Colonially nesting black-headed gulls (*Larus ridibundus*) had greater fledgling success because of lower predation than those atypical gulls with scattered nests (Patterson, 1965). Solitary nesting was clearly not adaptive, but it demonstrated a benefit of coloniality. Similarly, Craig's (1980) observation that pukeko (*Porphyrio porphyrio melanotus*) living in flocks fledged no young, seems to demonstrate that this unusual social system was maladaptive. It seems reasonable to refer to a variation which produces complete reproductive failure by the participants as 'pathological'. Dolhinow (1977) and Eisenberg (1981) have emphasized the possibility of truly pathological social behavior.

Sometimes intraspecific variation in social systems has been seen as adaptively neutral. Venables & Lack (1934, 1936), observing that great crested grebes (*Podiceps cristatus*) are sometimes territorial and sometimes colonial, argued that this variation demonstrated that neither system had any adaptive significance. Richard (1974) interpreted part of the variance observed in two populations of sifaka (*Propithecus verreauxi*) as an adaptively neutral outcome of local behavioral traditions.

The above approaches to social system variation tend to view it as noise obscuring the true signal. In some contexts, individual differences tend to be seen that way. However, individual differences, and the variations in social systems they sometimes produce, are often a clear signal that can reduce otherwise intractable noise in our understanding of social behavior.

1.3 VARIATION SEEN AS ADAPTIVE

Some authors have long recognized social system variation as a possible adaptive strategy. Feral domestic cats (*Felis domesticus*) exhibit complex and varying social interactions. They may be solitary or social (MacDonald *et al.*, 1987). Sometimes they decide priority via status differences; at other times the first animal present has priority (Leyhausen, 1965). Leyhausen suggested their flexibility offers a model for understanding variable social systems. The size and composition of social groups vary greatly in some species, especially small rodents, depending on the distribution of resources and population density. Eisenberg (1966) pointed out that small rodents characteristically have a high intrinsic reproductive potential and live in unpredictable environments. He suggested that for such species in such circumstances the 'plasticity' of 'loose' social organization could be an adaptive attribute. Crook (1970) identified intraspecific variation as a major feature of primate social organization. He pointed out its possible implications for understanding socioecology and proposed a tentative list of ecological variables that might act as determinants of social variation. Wilson (1975) discussed 'behavioral gradients' (primarily instances of intraspecific variation between dominance and territoriality) as adaptive adjustments to different circumstances.

Recognition of the significance of social system variation within species seems to be increasing rapidly. Bekoff *et al.* (1984) incorporated a section on such variation in their review of carnivores, and Moehlman (1989) devoted an entire review to intraspecific variation in canid social systems. Lott (1984) reviewed such variation in vertebrates and West-Eberhard (1989) reviewed instances of it in invertebrates in the general context of behavioral variation.

1.4 DEFINITION OF SOCIAL SYSTEMS

The view of social systems employed here follows Hinde (1976, 1983). Hinde identified a social organization as an outcome of a consistent set of social relationships. Social relationships, in turn, are the product of social interactions between individuals. By 'system' I will refer to the emergent outcome of a social relationship that seems to have a biological function. The form of mating relationships or care of offspring observed will be described as the mating system or parental care system. For example, when the interactions between golden-winged sunbirds take the form of each male attacking all male conspecifics within a particular area, but fleeing from all male conspecifics in other areas, the outcome is a territorial system. On the other hand, when each individual always supplants certain individuals, and always yields to certain other individuals wherever they are encountered, the emergent system is dominance. As in this example, alternative systems consist of the expression of mutually exclusive kinds of relationships. For example, animals cannot simultaneously be in both a territorial system and a dominance system, so those sets of relationships are mutually exclusive. Such categories are neither real nor immutable, but they do represent useful summaries of the current state of our knowledge and, therefore, are an appropriate starting point in extending it.

1.5   ANIMAL SOCIAL SYSTEMS THEORY BACKGROUND

Interest in the evolution of animal social systems as evolved phenomena has its roots in field studies of animal behavior. In the early decades of this century, social systems were described as part of general reports of the natural history or behavior of particular species, reported by field biologists (e.g., red deer (*Cervus elaphus*) (Darling, 1937), gibbons (*Hylobates lar*) (Carpenter, 1940), song sparrows (*Melospiza melodia*) (Nice, 1937)).

Most of these descriptions were not strongly guided by theory, although some addressed general issues; e.g., Howard (1920) was concerned with the relationship of territoriality to ecological issues. While conflicts of interest between individuals were certainly recognized, many instances of cooperative or care-giving behavior were implicitly or explicitly attributed to group selection (e.g., Wynne-Edwards, 1962).

In the mid-1960s several changes took place at about the same time. Workers began to interpret social systems as adaptive responses to ecological forces, including the type and distribution of food, predator pressure, and the plant community (e.g., Eisenberg, 1962, 1968; Crook, 1961, 1965). This track still continues and includes such landmark papers as Emlen & Oring's (1977) interpretation of mating systems as ecological adaptations.

An increasingly quantitative approach to theory and research in socioecology was stimulated by thinking such as Brown's (1964) analysis of territoriality. Brown showed that territoriality should occur when the benefits exceeded the costs. He predicted that it would occur in the middle ranges of resource availability.

New insight into cooperative and care-giving behavior was initiated by critiques of group selection (e.g., Lack, 1968; Williams, 1966) and the development of kinship selection theory by Hamilton (1964a,b). The implications of genetics for the evolution of social behavior were further revealed by theoretical analyses (including Trivers, 1972 and Alexander, 1974). These analyses emphasized the conflict in the genetic interests of mates and between them and their offspring, and they developed the implications of those conflicts for the evolved social systems. The conflict of interest between the sexes, for example, provides the evolutionary basis for the Evolutionarily Stable Strategy theory of mating systems (Maynard Smith, 1974, 1976, 1978).

1.6   CORRELATES AND DETERMINANTS OF INTRASPECIFIC VARIATION IN SOCIAL SYSTEMS

In many cases the alternatives appear to be adaptations to ecological, demographic and existing social system correlates. These correlates are often regarded as determinants. In some instances, experimental manipulations have demonstrated that they are. I will discuss these correlates as determinants even though that status is tentative in most cases. The ultimate determinants are discussed briefly in chapters 2 and 3 and more fully in chapter 4. There are at least four sorts of such determinants: ecological circumstances, demographics, kinship, and the prevailing pattern of social behavior. The role of these variables in determining social interactions and, hence, social systems, has been developed over several decades by hundreds of scientists. It is not possible to acknowledge the contribution each has made. However, I will be able to acknowledge a few of the central figures who have contributed to the development of the principal concepts as I discuss them in chapters 2, 3 and 4.

1.7   SOCIOECOLOGICAL ANALYSIS OF INTRASPECIFIC VARIATION IN SOCIAL SYSTEMS

Most reports of intraspecific variation have occurred in a conceptual environment strongly influenced by socioecology. Most recent analyses of such variation have naturally followed the approach of interspecific socioecology pioneered by Eisenberg (1962) and Crook (1965). In this approach the social system is analyzed as a mechanism for minimizing cost (usually in energy, risks of injury, or time spent) while maximizing benefits (ultimately in lifetime reproductive rate, but more immediately in energy gained, risk of predation reduced, etc.). A good fit between a set of ecological circumstances and a social system is explicitly or implicitly interpreted as an adaptation produced by natural selection.

Adaptiveness is currently the most frequently analyzed aspect of cases of intraspecific variation. Usually each social system is seen as the one best suited to the circumstances in which it is found. Spotted hyenas (*Crocuta crocuta*) on the Serengeti, for example, get most of their food by scavenging the remains of small, migratory prey. They are usually solitary and nomadic. Kruuk's (1972) interpretation of this pattern was that the food base on the Serengeti is usually too scanty and unpredictable to support large groups of hyenas or provide the energy required to defend territories. In contrast, most of the food in the Ngorongoro Crater is only available to groups large enough to kill it. Moreover, it is predictable and relatively abundant, so territorial defense seems both possible and functional. These hyenas are organized in large, cohesive social groups (clans) that defend territories all the year round (Kruuk, 1972). Kruuk argued that these different patterns are adaptive adjustments to different circumstances. This interpretation is supported by the fact that when prey density is unusually high on the Serengeti, the hyenas form small, temporary clans.

Such an economic analysis of alternative social systems is classical socioecology. However, classical socioecological analysis based on inter-specific comparisons usually assume that differences in social systems are the products of natural selection acting in the species' history. Thus there were territorial species and non-territorial species. But hyenas are territorial in some circumstances and not in others. In such cases the species is neither territorial nor non-territorial but can be either according to circumstances. The conceptual difference is important. While the economic analysis of the function of the behavior remains persuasive, to fully understand the occurrence of alternative social systems in the single species we must know the process that produces the observed alternations in behavior.

Crook (1989) and Dunbar (1988) pointed out that individual adjustments to optimize lifetime reproductive success are probably achieved via a number of interesting processes. Lott (1984) and Krebs & Davies (1987) argued that a complete understanding of (respectively) social system variation and optimization in behavioral ecology, generally requires knowledge of the proximate mechanisms involved.

1.8   THE MECHANICS OF SOCIAL SYSTEM VARIATION

Social system variation might be the result of (1) the social interactions of identical behavioral phenotypes in different circumstances, (2) the social interactions of different behavioral phenotypes in the same circumstances, or (3) the social interactions of different behavioral phenotypes in different circumstances.

In some cases it seems every individual (or at least every member of a particular age and sex class) does the same thing under all circumstances, and the varying social system is produced by varying circumstances. Three different mating systems (monogamy, polygyny, and polygynandry) in Red Sea damselfish (*Dascyllus aruanus*) seem to be produced directly by environmental variation with all individuals behaving the same way, but producing different outcomes according to the size of the coral heads on which they reside (Fricke, 1977) (see chapter 3).

However, in many cases change in social systems will be a consequence of change in social predispositions. An interesting historical note on hypothetical mechanisms is provided by von Haartman's (1951) suggestion that polyterritorial polygyny in pied flycatchers (*Ficedula hypoleuca*) is produced by appetitive behavior as the males seek a new place to sing songs no longer appropriate in the original territory. He goes on to note the greater reproductive success of polygynous males makes the evolution of polygyny understandable.

In fact, many instances of social system variation are the outcome of either populations or individuals interacting differently. One major difference among the forms of such variation is the time course of the changes. Caro & Bateson (1986) provided a scheme that classifies various routes to alternative states partially on the basis of their time course.

1.9   GENETIC DIFFERENCES BETWEEN POPULATIONS

In some cases generation after generation of different populations in different areas may manifest different social systems. Each social system could be the result of natural selection producing genetic differences between populations. Seghers (1974) has shown that the tendency of laboratory bred samples of guppies (*Poecilia reticulata*) from different populations to form schools is genetically determined. The populations most predisposed to form schools were from sections of a stream with more predators. Similarly, the young of chinook salmon (*Oncorhynchus tshawytscha*) spawning in small stream populations where territoriality was particularly adaptive were more aggressive than the young of salmon spawning in areas where territoriality was less beneficial (Taylor, 1988).

A number of psychological properties, or predispositions, have been demonstrated to have genetic correlates. Such predispositions seem likely to influence the social systems that interactions between individuals would produce. The amount of anxious behavior exhibited by rats and mice in open field tests can be related to genetic variation (Plomin *et al.*, 1980). The level of aggression in mice also has genetic heritability (Ebert & Hyde, 1976) as does the speed of acquisition of certain specific learning tasks (Bovet, 1977). In fact, heritability has been demonstrated for nearly all behavioral measures that have been tested (Hay, 1985). Covariation between behavioral traits and genetic differences are likely to act as determinants of social interactions, hence social relationships, and hence social systems. Unfortunately field data alone cannot demonstrate genetic influences. Evidence that different behavior is manifested by genetically isolated populations does not prove the behavioral difference is genetic. Different populations could have the same inclinations, but behave differently because their behavior was modified by different environmental circumstances.

1.10   MECHANISMS OPERATING WITHIN AN INDIVIDUAL'S LIFETIME

In other cases the population's social system changes from year to year. Few northern harriers (*Circus cyaneus*) breed polygynously in years of normal vole population density, but many more are polygynous in years of high vole numbers (Simmons *et al.*, 1986). Some mechanism must operate to make the individual behave one way in one year and differently in another year. In still other cases the social system changes from day to day or even from hour to hour. Sunbirds may have feeding territories in the morning, when the increased nectar in plants sequestered by territoriality contains enough energy to justify the costs of territoriality, but are dominance organized at other times of the day (Gill & Wolf, 1975; Wolf, 1978). The mechanism producing this shift may have only minutes to work (Lott & Lott, unpubl.).

These different interactions are produced by mechanisms. There must be two general kinds of mechanisms: those that produce an assessment of the individual organism's circumstances and those that change the individual's behavior. Some reports of intraspecific variation use an optimality approach, in essence arguing that if an alternative social system is better suited to the present circumstances (e.g., resource distribution) the animal will assess this difference and behave appropriately. This approach requires a mechanism to make the assessment and so raises the question of the nature of assessment mechanisms. Moreover, assessment by itself is not enough to produce change; there must also be a mechanism to implement the results of the assessment by appropriately altering the behavior. Most cigarette smokers have assessed their behavior pattern and found it less optimal than not smoking. But many of them have not shifted to that alternative. The behavior pattern persists in conflict with their assessment, because no behavioral mechanism sufficient to produce the change has operated.

Several mechanistic steps could be involved in a particular case of social system variation (Fig. 1.1). In many instances only some of these steps will be taken separately, with the rest incorporated in those. For example, some mechanisms may produce assessment and change simultaneously, e.g., genetic differences between populations.

Spotted hyenas illustrate these ideas. They live both in stable territorial clans and solitarily. Since the Serengeti population does both, we may assume it has been selected for flexibility. The assessment and change mechanisms might operate before adulthood via a predisposition set by nutrition, so that the social pattern was set by the time an individual became an adult, precluding all the following steps in Fig. 1.1. Alternatively, adult spotted hyenas may be socially plastic. If so, some or even all the mechanistic steps would occur before a particular social system would emerge. The number of steps will depend partly on the form the mechanisms take. If the mechanisms were highly cognitive and even 'conscious' (e.g. Griffin, 1984) all the represented steps would occur. If they were nutritional, hormonal, or followed a stimulus-response learning paradigm, assessment and change steps might be combined in a single process.

It is unlikely that any single mechanistic factor will account for a particular social system outcome (Caro & Bateson, 1986). All mechanistic processes are likely to interact with genetics and perhaps with each other, although one or another may be the primary factor in many cases.

There are many plausible but unproven mechanisms and hypothetical histories in this book. They are advanced primarily to illustrate conceptual issues and levels and potential points of attack on the question of the processes that produce variation in social systems.

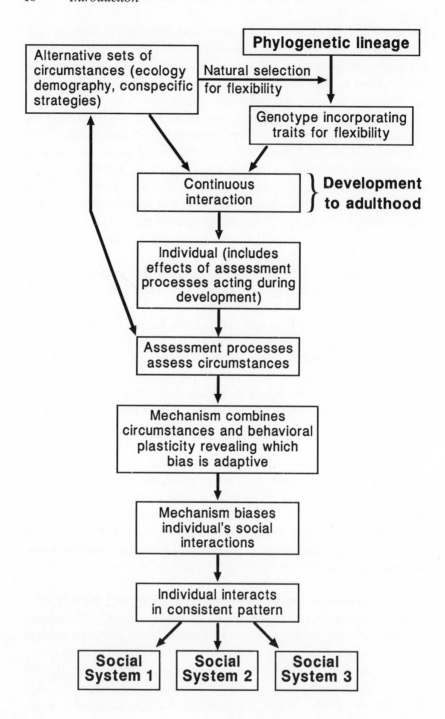

reports that might prove incorrect to the risk of excluding correct reports that might offer promising leads. My reasoning is that severe pruning at this stage could lead to the loss of some fruitful research directions.

We cannot make sense of the world without using some system of classification, and the one used in the preceding examples has proved useful. One way of looking at socioecology is that it has consisted largely of making sensible matches between an array of social systems and an array of ecological pressures and circumstances. This process depends on the current classification of social systems having useful biological reality, as it seems to have. Partly for this reason, and partly because the current literature assumes these definitions and is expressed in them, my review of that literature uses those categories. Useful though this set of categories is, some outcomes of social interactions are not well-represented in them. Perhaps work on changing social systems will stimulate development of additional ways to describe social systems.

1.17   VARIATIONS NOT REVIEWED

This review largely ignores the enormous amount of literature on alternative mating strategies and on group size. Alternative mating strategies are produced by qualitatively different social behavior, but the behavior tends to be consistent within a given morph or age class. For example, certain morphs or age classes defend territories or harems while other morphs or age classes breed opportunisticly. The focus here is on variations in relationships within the same age class or morph. The use of alternative mating strategies by different age classes or morphs has been extensively reviewed elsewhere, e.g., Howard (1978), Tutin (1979), Rubenstein (1980), Gross & Charnov (1980), Dunbar (1982), Gross (1982, 1983), Taborsky *et al.* (1986), and Hogg (1988). Instances of change in group size from one to two or more suggest a qualitative change in social interactions and so are reviewed, but I have not reviewed the more quantitative changes in size of groups of two or more.

2

Intraspecific variation in the distribution and relationship of individuals in space and time

2.1   GROUP MEMBERSHIP AS AN ALTERNATIVE TO SOLITARY LIVING

Individuals living solitarily are either neutral toward one another or repelled by one another. They ignore, attack or avoid conspecifics other than mates and offspring. In contrast, individuals living in groups are attracted to conspecifics and behave in ways that maintain proximity to at least some of them. Some instances of intraspecific variation from solitary to group membership are given in Table 2.1.

To describe or study group and solitary living as alternatives we must distinguish aggregations from groups and define group membership. Many studies of grouping behavior have relied on intuitive definitions of groups and never made the definitions explicit. When groups are operationally defined, groups of size one are included, so the smallest group has only one member. Being alone is usually operationally defined in terms of a relatively large distance between individuals and their attraction to or repulsion from one another. A second component of operational definitions of group membership includes the degree and form of interaction, the similarity or synchrony of behavior and sometimes similarity of orientation. This last criterion is used to indicate coordination of movement (Clutton-Brock *et al.*, 1982; Lott & Minta, 1983; Martin & Bateson, 1987). The most compelling example is in the similarity of orientation in schooling fish. The distinction between aggregations and groups is generally made on the basis of how long the individuals remain together, the number of different activities they engage in together and the degree to which their activities are integrated. The underlying idea is that group membership involves more than co-location, and the definitions seek to include behavioral indications that the animals adjust their behavior to maintain a cohesive group. For example, the presence of contact grunts

16

Table 2.1.   *Solitary and group as alternative social systems.*

Species	Differences in circumstances (S – when solitary, G – when grouped, NKD signifies no known difference in circumstances)	References
Spottail shiner *Notropis hudsonius*	NKD (alone when hungrier?)	Seghers, 1981
European-minnow *Phoxinus phoxinus*	G when minnow alarm substance present	Levesley & Magurran, 1988
Stickleback *Gasterosteus* spp.	More G when more ectoparasites	Poulin & Fitzgerald, 1989
Thalassoma bifasciatum	More G when more bottom irregularities	Mochek & Valdes-Munoz, 1983
Juvenile Atlantic salmon *Salmo salar*	In small aquaria, two roles: S dominant & dominated school	Keenleyside & Yamamoto, 1962
Coral trout *Plectropomus leopardus*	G in more exposed areas of reef	Goeden, 1978
Guppy *Poecilia reticulata*	G when predation pressure high	Seghers, 1974
Rainbow trout *Salmo gairdneri*	G in hatchery ponds, S when released; G in still water	Jenkins, 1971; Kalleberg, 1958
Sea trout *Salmo trutta*	G in still water	Kalleberg, 1958
Sockeye salmon fry *Oncorhynchus nerka*	Always G after experience with predator, sometimes S when naive	Ginetz & Larkin, 1976
Orange chromide cichlid *Etroplus maculatus*	G when threat of cannabalism high, S when threat lower	Ward & Samarakoon, 1981
Manini *Acanthrus triostegus*	G in areas of greater predation pressure & higher food competition	Barlow, 1974
Lavender tang *Acanthrus nigrofuscus*	G in areas where dominant species territorial	Barlow, 1974
Striped parrotfish *Scarus croicensis*	NKD	Ogden & Buckman, 1973; Robertson *et al.*, 1976
Spadefoot toad *Scaphiopus* spp.	G when food scarce (group swimming stirs bottom detritus)	Bragg, 1955

Table 2.1.   (*cont.*)

Species	Differences in circumstances (S – when solitary, G – when grouped, NKD signifies no known difference in circumstances)	References
Rio Grande turkey *Meleagris gallopavo*	G in open habitat, S in closed habitat	Watts & Stokes, 1971; Glazener, 1967; Smith, 1977; Balph *et al.*, 1980; Leopold, 1944
Wild × domestic turkey *Meleagris gallopavo*	Temporarily G after pen rearing, S in nature	Leopold, 1944
Common eider *Somateria mollisima*	G when gull predation higher	Munro & Bedard, 1977
Little blue heron *Egretta caerulea*	NKD	Caldwell, 1986
Great blue heron *Ardea herodias*	S when food widely scattered and/or easily defensible	Krebs, 1974
Pukeko *Porphyrio porphyrio melanotus*	NKD	Craig, 1979
Common tern *Sterna hirundo*	S when suitable shoreline available	Nisbet, 1983
Laughing gull *Larus atricilla*	G when stealing fish from terns	Hatch, 1975
Sanderling *Calidris alba*	NKD	Myers *et al.*, 1979a,b
Harris' hawk *Parabuteo unicinctus*	G where have large, elusive prey	Bednarz & Ligon, 1988
Blackshouldered kite *Elanus caeruleus*	G when food patchy and ephemeral	Mendelsohn, 1988
American goldfinch *Carduelis tristis*	NKD	Popp, 1986
Greenfinch *Carduelis chloris*	G when lower starvation risk	Ekman & Hake, 1988
Robin *Turdus migratorius*	NKD	Swann, 1975
Pied wagtail *Motacilla alba yarrellii*	G when food abundant	Davies, 1976
Magpie *Pica pica*	G when food clumped	Moller, 1983
House sparrow *Passer domesticus*	S when predation risk lower, temperature higher	Elgar, 1986

Table 2.1.   (*cont.*)

Species	Differences in circumstances (S – when solitary, G – when grouped, NKD signifies no known difference in circumstances)	References
Masked weaver *Ploceus heuglini*	NKD	Grimes, 1973
Euro kangaroo *Macropus robustus*	NKD	Ganslosser, 1980
Macropus greyi	S when in desert	Ganslosser, 1980
Grey kangaroo *Macropus fuliginosus*	NKD	Ganslosser, 1980
Eastern grey kangaroo *Macropus giganteus*	More often S when population less dense	Southwell, 1984
European rabbit *Oryctolagus cuniculus*	G when not enough burrows; G where soil permits digging of large burrows	Cowan & Bell, 1986; Roberts, 1987
Brown hare *Lepus europaeus*	S when food dispersed, G when food patchy	Monaghan & Metcalfe, 1985
Reedbuck *Redunca arundinum*	S in dense cover, G after fire destroyed cover	Jungius, 1971
Gemsbok *Oryx gazella*	S in dry season	Owens & Owens, 1984b
White-tailed deer *Odocoileus virginianus*	G in open habitat, S in closed habitat	Hardin *et al.*, 1976; Hirth, 1977
Roe deer *Capreolus capreolus*	S when less food, more cover	Maublanc *et al.*, 1987
Burro *Equus asinus*	G when food abundant, S where food sparse	R. Rudman, pers. comm.
Red fox *Vulpes vulpes*	NKD	Kolb, 1986
Coyote *Canis latrans*	G when large carrion being defended by pairs or packs; G when aggregations overwhelm defense; G when prey large and clumped; G when hunting deer, & when deer more vulnerable	Camenzind, 1978; Bowen, 1981; Bekoff & Wells, 1980; Bowyer, 1987
Wolf *Canis lupus*	S where large prey scarce	van Haaften *et al.*, 1983
Golden jackal *Canis aureus*	Pairs when food distributed, packs when concentrated	MacDonald, 1979
Spotted hyena *Crocata crocata*	S when prey small, migratory often scarce, G when prey large, dense & non-migratory	Kruuk, 1972

Table 2.1.   (*cont.*)

Species	Differences in circumstances (S – when solitary, G – when grouped, NKD signifies no known difference in circumstances)	References
Brown hyena *Hyaena brunnea*	G when food (& intraspecific competition) greater; G when larger carrion available	Skinner, 1976; Owens & Owens, 1978; 1979a,b
Striped hyena *Hyaena hyaena*	G when food patchy	Kruuk, 1976; MacDonald, 1978
Cheetah *Acinonyx jubatus*	NKD; G when more males in litter	Frame & Frame, 1981; Caro & Collins, 1986, 1987
Lion *Panthera leo*	S in dry season	Owens & Owens, 1984b
Domestic cat *Felis domesticus*	G when food abundant, clumped	MacDonald *et al.*, 1987
Long-tailed macaque *Macaca fascicularis*	Large subadult males often S in main fruiting season	van Schaik & van Noordwijk, 1986
Red-backed voles *Clethrionomys* spp.		Viitala, 1980
Grey-sided vole *Clethrionomys rufocanus*	G where heat loss greater	Ylonen & Viitala, 1987
Meadow vole *Microtus agrestis*	G when neighbors more familiar	Viitala, 1977, 1980
Vole *Microtus arvalis*	G when population density increases	Frank, 1957
Taiga vole *Microtus xanthognathus*	G in winter	Wolff & Lidicker, 1981
Norway rat *Rattus norvegicus*	S when food scarce	Izumi, 1973
European badger *Meles meles*	S when fewer earthworms	Kruuk, 1986; Kruuk & Parish, 1982, 1987
Harbour seal *Phoca vitulina*	G when found at haul-out sites	DaSilva & Terhune, 1988
Southern sea lion *Otaria byronia*	G to overcome defense of mating territory	Campagna *et al.*, 1988

could be a defining attribute. The operational definition for a particular species will depend on knowledge of that species ethogram. However, in practice, individuals are often recorded as members of groups because they meet some proximity criterion. This may be justified by previously finding that members of this species close to one another interact and maintain proximity.

2.2   GROUP VERSUS SOLITARY LIVING: background

Group life has several costs: group members compete for food and shelter and may burden one another with diseases and parasites (Alexander, 1974; Bertram, 1978). There are also several benefits. One of the most important is that group membership is a way of countering predator pressure.

Group living animals suffer less predation than solitary individuals (e.g., Page & Whiteacre, 1975; Kenward, 1978). Group members lower the predator pressure on themselves in several ways. One way is by spotting predators sooner. Powell (1974) and Lazarus (1979) have shown that birds in a flock are aware of a predator's approach before solitary birds. Sometimes there is active group defense. Musk oxen (*Ovibos moschatus*) form a defense circle facing outward when attacked by wolves (*Canis lupus*) (Tener, 1954, 1965). Group members may attack a predator *en masse* (mobbing). Ground squirrels (*Spermophilus beldingi*) mob non-poisonous snakes (Owings & Coss, 1977), and flycatchers mob woodpeckers and squirrels (Curio, 1975).

Group members sometimes seem to confuse the predator by fleeing erratically or explosively. Neill & Cullen (1974) showed that several aquatic predators made fewer captures per attack when attacking schools of prey fish as compared to attacking solitary members of the same species. Members of groups may also avoid predation by maneuvering to increase the chance that another group member will be taken by the predator (Williams, 1964; Hamilton, 1971).

Predators may also benefit from group membership by increasing their rate of prey capture or defense of a resource. This is the most convincing explanation of sociality in social carnivores (Gittleman, 1989). Groups of wild dogs (*Lycaon pictus*) capture prey that individuals could not capture (Frame & Frame, 1981). Coyotes (*Canis latrans*) hunt in groups when preying on mule deer (*Odocoileus hemionus*) (Bowen, 1981). Harris' hawks (*Parabuteo unicinctus*) hunt jackrabbits (*Lepus californicus*) cooperatively. Groups of five or six were much more successful than smaller numbers (Bednarz, 1988).

Carcasses may be better defended by groups than by individuals. Packer (1986) proposed that sociality evolved in African lions (*Panthera leo*) to facilitate retention of carcasses, and Bekoff & Wells (1980) report that coyotes feeding on large carrion (e.g. elk (*Cervus elaphus canadensis*) carcasses) facultatively form groups.

Finally, group members may be harassed less than solitary individuals when foraging in an area defended by a territorial conspecific or similar competitor. Barlow (1974) has shown that grouped manini, a surgeon fish (*Acanthrus triostegus*), are harassed less than solitary individuals under those circumstances. Myers *et al.* (1979b) demonstrated the same effect in sanderlings (*Calidris alba*).

2.3   ECOLOGICAL DETERMINANTS OF GROUP AND SOLITARY LIVING AS ALTERNATIVES

Higher predator pressure is associated with the occurrence of group living as an alternative to solitary living in many species. Guppies are small freshwater fish that feed on small invertebrates. Small fish may have many predators, creating some pressure to live in groups. But conspecifics usually compete for food, which imposes a cost of group foraging. Their optimal degree of predisposition to live in groups should balance the benefits of avoiding predation against the costs of foraging competition. In a now classic paper, Seghers (1974) demonstrated genetic differences in the predisposition of individuals from two populations to form groups and showed those differences should be adaptive in the different environments of the two populations.

In Trinidad, guppies inhabit most of a single stream. The downstream population is prey to a predatory fish in the same community, but a waterfall has proven an impassible barrier to this predator so the population above the waterfall is free of it. In nature the downstream population tends to form groups, while individuals from above the waterfall are more likely to be solitary. Guppies taken from the stream and placed in aquaria differ in the same way, and their aquarium-born offspring also behave as their respective ancestors did (Seghers, 1974).

Manini experiencing increased contact with predators no longer graze alone in their coral-reef habitat but form foraging groups (Barlow, 1974). Group living, as an alternative to solitary living, also appears in many species when they occupy more open habitat even if former predators are no longer present. White-tailed deer (*Odocoileus virginianus*) are solitary in most areas, but populations living in open habitat where they are more vulnerable to wolves and coyotes tend to form groups (Hirth, 1977). Seghers, Barlow and Hirth all suggest that group living reduces the risk of predation but increases the level of food competition, and that the alternative social systems of these species are adjustments to the relative intensity of these ecological demands.

Certain forms of competition over food are associated with group rather than solitary living. Manini excluded from the territories of individuals of a dominant species in their guild form large aggregations that overwhelm territorial defense and feed in the otherwise defended space (Barlow, 1974). Solitary coyotes attracted to a large unit of carrion but denied access to it by an established pair or pack may form temporary, mutually tolerant aggregations that displace the defenders (Camenzind, 1978).

Groups sometimes form when individuals cannot capture the available prey. Coyotes occupying mule deer habitat have been observed living in packs which kill adult deer that individuals could not kill (Bowen, 1981; Bowyer, 1987). Spadefoot toad (*Scaphiopus*) tadpoles usually forage solitarily, but when food is scarce in the water column they sometimes swim in large groups. The hydraulic effect of their mass swimming brings detritus from the bottom of the shallow ponds into the water column where the tadpoles can feed on it (Bragg, 1955). Barlow, Camenzind, Bowen, Bowyer and Bragg all suggest that these aggregations function to make otherwise inaccessible food obtainable.

2.4 COLONIALITY, LEKKING, ALL-PURPOSE TERRITORY, UNDEFENDED HOME RANGES, DOMINANCE, DESPOTISM, AND FLOCKING-SCHOOLING AS ALTERNATIVE SPACING SYSTEMS

Spacing systems describe the pattern of distribution of a species in space and time. They also describe the social processes by which resources are allocated among the members of a population. Alternating between different spacing systems often seems to be a way of adjusting to the levels of several kinds of ecological and demographic pressures that interact in sometimes complicated ways.

Four of the seven spacing systems considered in this section involve site-specific aggressive interactions and site-specific dominance. The social systems produced by these interactions differ as follows: individuals occupying all-purpose territories have site-specific relationships both in the area where they breed and in the area where they feed. In contrast, lekking or colonial individuals have site-specific relationships only in the area where they breed. The all-purpose territory holders have site-specific dominance in all or most of their home range. In lekking and colonial systems individuals have such dominance in only part of their home range. Reports of a single species living in more than one of these alternative systems are aggregated in Tables 2.2 through to 2.7. Apparently, lekking or colonial individuals are stimulated to aggression by an out-group conspecific in only part of their home range.

In populations organized by dominance, despotism or flocking-schooling, individuals or units have overlapping home ranges. Their relationships are determined by location-independent interactions. Territorial, colonial, and lekking animals are stimulated to aggress or yield by the location of the animal with which they are interacting. Individuals in populations organized by dominance or despotism are stimulated to aggression or submission by which two individuals interact, rather than where they are. The systems differ in the degree of ranking of individuals among themselves. Territorial and flocking-schooling individuals are all at one rank, while dominance organized individuals are all at different ranks (or at least all have dominant – subordinate relationships within each dyad). In populations organized by despotism one is dominant to the others which are all of equal rank.

2.5   TERRITORIALITY: background

Howard (1920) recognized that territoriality functioned to control access to resources, notably forage. Others have extended this insight to include other resources, such as display areas (Lack, 1968) and access to mates (Emlen, 1978).

As the number of functions of territoriality grew, the generality of the concept shrank. Conceptual generality was restored by Brown (1964) who aggregated all these functions by labeling them benefits, and proposed that whenever the benefits of territoriality (whatever form they took) exceeded its costs (such as time, energy and increased risk of injury or predation) territoriality would be favourably selected. Cost and benefits were converted to the same coin by defining both in terms of their contribution to lifetime fitness.

Brown's work helped structure empirical studies and clarified their goals, and his concepts remain central to the thinking about territoriality today. However, applying these concepts in empirical studies is often difficult. Lifetime fitness is often hard to determine, particularly in long-

Table 2.2. *Territoriality and coloniality as alternative social systems.*

Species	Differences in circumstances (T – when territorial, C – when colonial, NKD signifies no known difference in circumstances)	References
Great crested grebe *Podiceps cristatus*	C when higher predation pressure?	McCartan & Simmons, 1956
Black swan *Cygnus atratus*	C on islands, T in wetland patches	Braithwaite, 1981
Mute swan *Cygnus olor*	NKD	Bloch, 1970; Bacon, 1980
Mallard *Anas platyrhynchos*	C when nesting habitat limited (are mallards T elsewhere?)	Browne *et al.*, 1983
South Polar skua *Catharacta maccormicki*	Same habitat & food, Trillmich believes C's in marginal area (failed T's)	Trillmich, 1978
Arctic skua *Stercorarius parasiticus*	T feeding on lemmings, C when kleptoparasitic on piscivorous seabirds	Pitelka *et al.*, 1955; Andersson & Gotmark, 1980
Brown-hooded gull *Larus maculipenis*	NKD	Burger, 1974
Osprey *Pandion haliaetus*	More C in coastal habitats	Greene, 1987
Smooth-billed ani *Crotophaga ani*	T when abundant, C when rare	Davis, 1941
Silky-throated flycatcher *Phainopepla nitens*	T feeding on plant with long fruiting season, C on plant with short fruiting season	Walsberg, 1977, 1978
Fieldfare *Turdus pilaris*	NKD – C alternates with solitary, possibly T	Wiklund, 1982
Australian magpie *Gymnorhina tibicen*	NKD	Carrick, 1963
Northern oriole *Icterus galbula*	T when food at higher density	Pleasants, 1979
Yellow-hooded black-bird *Agelaius icterocephalus*	C when lived in area of higher 1) nest parasitism, 2) nest predation, 3) food abundance	Wiley & Wiley, 1980a

lived vertebrates. Consequently, most studies substitute shorter term indices of fitness such as offspring in a season or increased forage availability.

Frequently, however, it is hard to compare costs and benefits using

Table 2.3.   *Territoriality and lekking as alternative social systems.*

Species	Differences in circumstances (T – when territorial, L – when lek forming, NKD signifies no known difference in circumstances)	References
Queen parrotfish *Scarus vetula*	NKD	Clavijo, 1983
Bullfrog *Rana catesbeiana*	May L when population more dense	Ryan, 1980
Blue grouse *Dendragapus obscurus*	Both T & L in previously logged forest, T only in unlogged forest	Blackford, 1958, 1963 (but see Lewis, 1985); Bendell, 1955
Buff-breasted sandpiper *Tryngites subruficollis*	T when nest habitat scarce, defendable	Cartar & Lyon, 1988
Topi *Damiliscus korrigum*	T in less dense population, more wooded environment, L on open plains; NKD	Monfort-Brahm, 1975; Duncan, 1975; Gosling, 1987; Gosling *et al.*, 1987
Uganda kob *Adenota kob*	Both T & L in more dense population, L only in less dense population & more grazers	Leuthold, 1966
Lechwe *Kobus leche*	T when habitat not flooded, L when flooding produces crowding on remaining land	Robbel & Child, 1975; Schuster, 1976
Fallow deer *Dama dama*	NKD	Clutton-Brock *et al.*, 1988

short term indices because they are in such different forms. How can one know if costs measured in increased risk of predation are greater or less than benefits measured in increased forage availability?

This problem is substantially smaller in studies of nectarivorous birds. The major cost of territoriality – the extra energy spent in territorial defense – can be determined by constructing time-energy budgets and expressed in calories. The benefit of foraging territoriality – increased nectar in the flowers defended by territorial behavior – can be measured directly and also expressed in calories. Consequently a strong test of Brown's predictions is possible in this system. Many studies of territoriality have exploited this model, and several have studied its implications

Table 2.4. *Territoriality and undefended home ranges as alternative social systems.*

Species	Differences in circumstances (T – when territorial, UHR – when have undefended home range, NKD signifies no known difference in circumstances)	References
Striped parrotfish *Scarus croicensis*	NKD	Ogden & Buckman, 1973; Robertson *et al.*, 1976
Threespine stickleback *Gasterosteus aculeatus*	More T when fewer females	Pressley, 1981
Rainbow trout *Salmo gairdneri*	T in faster flows, less dense population; UHR in still water	Cole & Noakes, 1980; Newman, 1956
Eastern brook trout *Salvelinus fontinalis*	UHR in still water	Newman, 1956
Char *Salmo alpinus*	Females T when few male territories	Fabricius & Gustafson, 1953
Atlantic salmon *Salmo salar*	T when water velocity higher	Kalleberg, 1958
Sea trout *Salmo trutta*	T when water velocity higher	Kalleberg, 1958
Pygmy sunfish *Elassoma evergladei*	T when prey clumped, or prey dispersed & population density mid-range	Rubenstein 1981b
Ayu-fish *Plecoglossus altivelis*	NKD	Kawanabe, 1972
Tilapia *Oreochromis mossambicus*	NKD	Munro & Singh, 1987
Pukeko *Porpyrio porphyrio melanotus*	T where food & cover more patchy	Craig, 1979
Great crested grebe *Podiceps cristatus*	NKD	Venables & Lack, 1934, 1936
Great blue heron *Ardea herodius*	Food T when feeding on rodents, UHR when feeding in intertidal (colonial nesting)	Krebs, 1974
Common tern *Sterna hirundo*	T where suitable shoreline available	Nisbet, 1983
Sanderling *Calidris alba*	T when food sources concentration high & intruder pressure not too high; UHR when intruder pressure high	Connors *et al.*, 1981

Table 2.4.   (*cont.*)

Species	Differences in circumstances (T – when territorial, UHR – when have undefended home range, NKD signifies no known difference in circumstances)	References
Acorn woodpecker *Melanerpes formicivorous*	UHR when acorn crop poor	Hannon *et al.*, 1987
Mousebird *Colius striatus*	NKD	Decoux, 1982
Iwi *Vestiaria coccinae*	T when nectar production moderate, UHR when production high or low	Carpenter & MacMillen, 1976
Rufous hummingbird *Selasehorus rufus*	T when food widely distributed & population low, UHR when food concentrated & population high	Kodric-Brown & Brown, 1978
Pied wagtail *Motacilla alba yarrellii*	T when feeding predictably good but defensible	Davies, 1976
Fieldfare *Turdus pilaris*	T when food abundant & patchy	Tye, 1986
Townsend's solitaire *Myadestes townsendi*	T when food normal for area, UHR when food scarce	Lederer, 1981
Yellow-faced grassquit *Tiaris olivacea*	T when suitable habitat continuous?	Pulliam *et al.*, 1972
Blackbird *Turdus merula*	T in lower population density, UHR when T population experiences severe winter freeze	Steinbacher, 1953; Snow, 1956
Brown-headed cowbird *Molothrus ater*	UHR where feed among grazing ungulates; T where host nests abundant	Elliott, 1980; Duffy, 1982
Burro *Equus asinus*	T when food abundant, UHR when food low; T elsewhere, UHR in central Australia; T where food abundant and patchy, UHR where food dispersed and sparse	Woodward, 1979; Hoffmann, 1983; R. Rudman, pers. comm.
Feral horse *Equus caballus*	UHR on Exmoor, T elsewhere; T in more productive, easier defended range; T elsewhere, UHR in central Australia	Gates, 1979; Rubenstein, 1981a; Hoffmann, 1983

Table 2.4. *(cont.)*

Species	Differences in circumstances (T – when territorial, UHR – when have undefended home range, NKD signifies no known difference in circumstances)	References
Pronghorn *Antilocapra americana*	T when hunting pressure lower	Copeland, 1980
Topi *Damiliscus korrigum*	NKD	Estes, 1966
Okavanga lechwe *Kobus leche leche*	T in confined habitat, UHR in open habitat	Lent, 1969
Impala *Aepyceros melampus*	UHR when population density high?	Warren, 1974
Mule deer *Odocoileus hemionus*	T when food more abundant/ more patchy	Miller, 1974; Geist, 1981
Roe deer *Capreolus capreolus*	T in more productive habitat	Prior, 1968
Bobcat *Lynx rufus*	T when population lower, age structure lower	Zezulak & Schwab, 1979
Cheetah *Acinonyx jubatus*	More T when in coalitions	Caro & Collins, 1986
Lion *Panthera leo*	UHR in dry season	Owens & Owens, 1984b
Spotted hyena *Crocata crocata*	T when population high, prey large & sedentary	Kruuk, 1972
Brown hyena *Hyaena brunnea*	T when food abundant, UHR when food scarce	Skinner, 1976; Owens & Owens, 1979a,b
Coyote *Canis latrans*	NKD	Bekoff & Wells, 1980; Bowen, 1981; Camenzind, 1978
Grey wolf *Canis lupus*	T when feed on non-migratory prey, UHR when feed on migratory prey	Mech, 1970; Peterson, 1979; Miller, 1979
Red fox *Vulpes vulpes*	NKD	Kolb, 1986
Black-backed jackal *Canis mesomelas*	UHR in dry season	Owens & Owens, 1979?
European rabbit *Oryctolagus cuniculus*	UHR when females do not group	Cowan & Bell, 1986

Table 2.4.   (*cont.*)

Species	Differences in circumstances (T – when territorial, UHR – when have undefended home range, NKD signifies no known difference in circumstances)	References
Desert woodrat *Neotoma lepida*	T when no avian predators, UHR with avian predators	Bleich & Schwartz, 1975; Vaughn & Schwartz, 1980
Allegheny woodrat *Neotoma floridana*	T when shelter limited but food not, communal when food limited but shelter not	Kinsey, 1977
Subarctic vole *Microtus agrestis*	T more often in grassland than forest	Viitala, 1977, 1980
California vole *Microtus californicus*	Females less T when abundant food clumped	Ostfeld, 1986
House mouse *Mus musculus*	T when population density high, UHR when population low	Mihok, 1979
Red squirrel *Tamiasciurus hudsonicus*	T in forest, UHR when on campus with other squirrel species present	Smith, 1968; Layne, 1954
River otter *Lutra lutra*	T on streams & lakes, UHR on sea coast	Erlinge, 1967, 1968; Kruuk & Hewson, 1978; MacDonald & Mason, 1980
European badger *Meles meles*	Less T when earthworms less abundant	Kruuk & Parish, 1987
Sifaka *Propithecus verreauxi*	NKD	Richard, 1974

for intraspecific variation in social systems (e.g., Gill & Wolf, 1975; Carpenter & MacMillen, 1976).

2.6   DOMINANCE: background

It often happens that one individual consistently has priority over another in access to some resource such as food, water or mating opportunities. Frequently, this dominant individual has priority of access to several resources, making the outcome of many interactions predictable by

Table 2.5.   *Territoriality and dominance hierarchies as alternative social systems.*

Species	Differences in circumstances (T – when territorial, D – when dominance organized, NKD signifies no known difference in circumstances)	References
Rainbow trout *Salmo gairdneri*	T when feeding stations much more productive, D when difference is small; T in stream, D in pool	Jenkins, 1969; Newman, 1956; Cole & Noakes, 1980
Char *Salmo alpinus*	Females T when few male territories	Fabricius & Gustafson, 1953
Green sunfish *Lepomis cyanellus*	T in aquaria most often when barriers divided space	Greenberg, 1947
Pumpkinseed sunfish *Lepomis gibbosus*	NKD	Erickson, 1967
Pygmy sunfish *Elassoma evergladei*	T when prey clumped & dispersed and population density mid-range	Rubenstein, 1981a
Chuckwalla *Sauromalus obesus*	T in years with annual plant growth, D with only few patches of perennial plants	Berry, 1974
Arizona chuckwalla *Sauromalus obesus tumidus*	T when less crowded	Prieto & Ryan, 1978
Lizard *Anolis aeneus*	NKD	Stamps, 1973
Lizard *Liocephalus carinatus coryi*	T when uncrowded	Evans, 1953
Chicken *Gallus gallus*	T uncrowded, D crowded	McBride *et al.*, 1969
Pukeko *Porphyrio porphyrio melanotus*	T where food & cover more patchy	Craig, 1979
Sage grouse *Centrocercus urophasianus*	D when late snow obscures landmarks; D when male display begins before territories established	Gibson & Bradbury, 1987
Sanderling *Calidris alba*	T when intruder pressure not too high	Myers, *et al.*, 1979a,b
Iwi *Vestiaria coccinea*	T when nectar content lower	Carpenter & MacMillan, 1976
Golden-winged sunbird *Nectarinia reichenowi*	T when nectar production moderate, D when nectar production high or low	Gill & Wolf, 1975

Table 2.5.   (*cont.*)

Species	Differences in circumstances (T – when territorial, D – when dominance organized, NKD signifies no known difference in circumstances)	References
Wagtail *Motacilla alba alba*	D when confined in small space	Zahavi, 1971
Red-winged blackbird *Agelaius phoeniceus*	NKD	Hurley & Robertson, 1984
Pine siskin *Cardaelis pinus*	T when food patchy	Balph & Balph, 1979
House mouse *Mus musculus*	T more common when resources concentrated, D when resources very dispersed or population very crowded; D when first colonize new area	Bronson, 1979; Crowcroft, 1955; Davis, 1958; Anderson & Hill, 1965; Wolff, 1985
Meadow vole *Microtus agrestis*	More T when neighbors less familiar	Viitala, 1977, 1980
Woodrat *Neotoma fuscipes*	D when more crowded	Kinsey, 1971
Woodchuck *Marmota monax*	T where low population density, D where high population density	Ferron & Ouellet, in press
Allegheny woodrat *Neotoma floridana magister*	T where shelter sparse	Kinsey, 1977
Hippopotamus *Hippopotamus amphibius*	T when river flow filling deep pools for all large males	Karstad & Hudson, 1986
Feral ass *Equus asinus*	T in rich patch of resources	Woodward, 1979
Pronghorn *Antilocapra americana*	T when undisturbed, D when disrupted by heavy hunting, have low density food supply; D when no older male cohort	Bromley, 1969; Kitchen, 1974; Copeland, 1980; Byers & Kitchen, 1988
Grant's gazelle *Gazella granti*	T with more abundant food, dominion with less food	Walther, 1972
Impala *Aepyceros melampus*	T with lower population density, longer breeding season	Warren, 1974; Jarman, 1979; Jarman & Jarman, 1974
Lechwe *Kobus leche leche*	T where habitat limited	Lent, 1969

Table 2.5.   (*cont.*)

Species	Differences in circumstances (T – when territorial, D – when dominance organized, NKD signifies no known difference in circumstances)	References
White-tailed deer *Odocoileus virginanus*	More T when older buck cohort present & sex ratio nearer to 1	Marchinton & Atkeson, 1985

Table 2.6.   *Territoriality and despotism as alternative social systems.*

Species	Differences in circumstances (T – when territorial, DES – when despotic, NKD signifies no known difference in circumstances)	References
Atlantic salmon *Salmo salar*	T when enough space for all, DES when group in space large enough for only one territory	Keenlyside & Yamamoto, 1962
Arctic char *Salmo alpinus*	T when space for all, DES when in space large enough for only one territory	Fabricius & Gustafson, 1953
Arizona chuckwalla *Sauromalus obesus*	T when uncrowded, DES when crowded	Prieto & Ryan, 1978; Berry, 1974
Black lizard *Ctenosaura pectisecta*	T when uncrowded, DES when crowded	Evans, 1951
Lizard *Liocephalus carinatus coryi*	T when uncrowded, DES when crowded	Evans, 1953
Black rat *Rattus rattus*	T when uncrowded, DES when crowded	Barnett, 1958
Norway rat *Rattus norvegicus*	T when uncrowded, DES when crowded	Barnett, 1958
House mouse *Mus musculus*	T in moderate densities, DES in high densities when cannot escape; NKD	Anderson, 1961; Hurst, 1987

Table 2.7. *Territoriality and schooling-flocking as alternative social systems.*

Species	Differences in circumstances (T – when territorial, SF – when school or flock, NKD signifies no known difference in circumstances)	References
Striped parrotfish *Scarus croicensis*	NKD	Ogden & Buckman, 1973; Buckman & Ogden, 1973; Robertson *et al.*, 1976
Atlantic salmon fry *Salmo salar*	T when in running water; in area with longer time exposure to fluctuation or reduction in prey, many stop T	Kalleberg, 1958; Symons, 1973, 1974
Atlantic salmon smolts *Salmo salar*	S-F when migrating, T when migration blocked	Kalleberg, 1958
Sanderling *Calidris alba*	T when prey density moderate, S-F when prey density high or low or predators in general area	Myers, *et al.*, 1979a,b, 1981; Connors, pers. comm.
Buff-breasted sandpiper *Tryngites subruficollis*	F when predator present	Myers, 1980
Pukeko *Porphyrio porphyrio*	All breed T, open habitat foragers, S-F when not breeding	Craig, 1979
White wagtail *Motacilla alba alba*	T when food clumped	Zahavi, 1971
Pied wagtail *Motacilla alba*	F when little food in foraging territory	Davies & Houston, 1983
Brown-headed cowbird *Molothrus ater*	T at mid-range density	Rothstein *et al.*, 1984
Magpie *Pica pica*	Gather when habitat saturated	Birkhead & Clarkson, 1985
Yellow-faced grassquit *Tiaris olivacea*	T when suitable habitat continuous	Pulliam *et al.*, 1972
Reedbuck *Redunca arundinum*	T in closed (normal) habitat, S-F when fire eliminates cover or water holes dry up & individuals concentrate	Jungius, 1971

observation of only a few. This makes dominance a powerful organizational principle for animal social systems. At times it was relied on so heavily that its role in structuring social relations was exaggerated. The critics such as Rowell (1974) and Bernstein (1976) pointed out that an animal dominant in competition for one resource may be subordinate in competition for another, that a strongly motivated subordinate may reverse the usual outcome of competition for a particular resource. They also noted that many studies of dominance used crowded, captive animals where the level of aggression and hence the role of dominance was exaggerated. These criticisms are well taken, but dominance remains an important concept to students of social systems. For example, Dewsbury (1982) has reviewed a large literature showing that dominant males have more offspring in a wide range of species.

When resources are not distributed by territoriality, they are often distributed by dominance. Intraspecific variation in which system organizes a particular population at particular times is common (see Table 2.5).

2.7   ECOLOGICAL DETERMINANTS OF COLONIALITY AND TERRITORIALITY AS ALTERNATIVES

Predictably located food resources are associated with all-purpose territories in some species that are colonial when feeding from unpredictable food sources. Nesting parasitic jaegers (*Stercorarius parasiticus*) feeding on lemmings (*Lemmus lemmus*) establish all-purpose territories (Fig. 2.1). In contrast, conspecifics in the same general area feeding on fish taken kleptoparasitically from other sea birds, nest colonially (Pitelka *et al.*, 1955; Andersson & Gotmark, 1980). Since they steal the fish immediately after it is captured from wide-ranging schools of marine fish, the location of their food supply is unpredictable.

In other cases, the suitability of the area of available food for nesting may determine whether a colonial or an all-purpose pattern is used. South Polar skuas (*Catharacta maccormicki*) feeding in an area with suitable nest sites defended both at an all purpose territory centered on the nest, while individuals excluded from that feeding area nested colonially and travelled to feed (Trillmich, 1978). The colonial pattern produced fewer young than the first, and Trillmich suggested that it was merely the best of the options remaining to skuas unable to establish themselves in better areas. A limited nesting habitat is sometimes correlated with coloniality in birds that would otherwise be territorial.

Black swans (*Cygnus atratus*) are colonial on islands where nesting space is limited, but territorial in less limited wetland patches (Braithwaite, 1981).

Sometimes coloniality seems to offer the ecological advantage of using the other members of the colony as sources of information. Krebs (1974) and Walsberg (1977) have suggested that colonial nesting may facilitate the discovery of unpredictable food sources since it permits birds to follow one another. That would be advantageous when the information available from conspecifics outweighed the loss of food to those same conspecifics as competitors. Greene (1987) reported such a situation in osprey (*Pandion haliaetus*). The normally territorial osprey nested in a colony. They were feeding on both schooling and non-schooling fish and observed each other returning to the nest with fish. When the returning bird was carrying a fish from a schooling species, the osprey retraced that bird's flight path and searched for fish from the same school. When the returning bird carried a fish of a solitary species the neighbors did not retrace its flight path. This appears to be generally advantageous. The schooling fish were in such large schools that the osprey did not compete

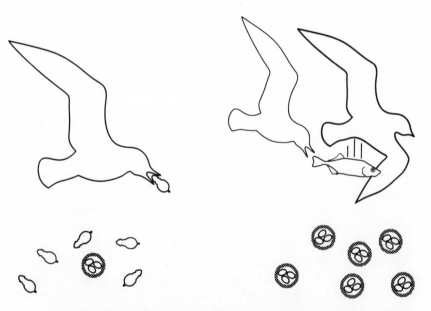

Fig. 2.1. Parasitic jaeger social system adjusts to the lemming population. Jaegers feeding on lemmings are territorial when lemmings are abundant, but when lemmings are scarce the jaegers feed kleptoparasitically from other sea birds.

with one another, but they were a useful source of information for each other.

Intense predation or nest parasitism is sometimes associated with either colonial nesting or all-purpose territories depending upon the species' antipredator behavior. The yellow-hooded blackbird (*Agelaius icterocephalus*), which has a mobbing antipredator behavior, lives in APTs when predator pressure is low and colonially when predator pressure is high (Wiley & Wiley, 1980a,b). In contrast, great crested grebes, which have a cryptic antipredator strategy, are more likely to be spaced in all-purpose territories if predator pressure is high, but colonial if it is low (McCartan & Simmons, 1956). It is noteworthy that the value of colonial or solitary nesting may vary greatly from predator to predator. Black-headed gulls preyed upon by foxes and carrion crows (*Corvus corone*) had higher nest success in colonies (Patterson, 1965). On the other hand, brown-hooded gulls (*Larus maculipenis*) preyed upon by caracaras (*Polyborus plancus*) had greater nest success when nesting solitarily (Burger, 1974). (This example is developed further in chapter 6.)

2.8   DETERMINANTS OF LEKKING AND TERRITORIALITY AS ALTERNATIVES

Variations in population density are correlated with lekking and APTs as alternative spacing systems. Topi (*Damaliscus lunatus korrigum*), Uganda Kob (*Kobus kob thomasi*) and lechwe (*Kobus lechwe*) all lek at high population densities and hold APTs at lower densities (Monfort-Brahm, 1975; Duncan, 1975; Leuthold, 1966; Robbel & Child, 1975; Schuster, 1976). Lekking may develop from territoriality when a high population density produces so much intruder pressure that larger spaces are not defensible. For example, topi in Akagera Park in Rwanda, lek in grassy meadows where lion predation appears to be lower, and females come in large numbers at evening to spend the night (Monfort-Brahm, pers. comm.; Lott, unpubl. obs.). Gosling (1990) proposed this analysis of the ecological determination of lekking in topi in the Masai Mara in Kenya.

2.9   DETERMINANTS OF TERRITORY, UNDEFENDED HOME RANGE AND DOMINANCE AS ALTERNATIVES

Brown (1964) predicted that economic defensibility of food resources would be a major determinant of interspecific differences in territoriality. An undefended home range as an alternative to territoriality is most commonly observed when the distribution or availability of, or competition for, food changes its defensibility as a resource. The iwi (*Vestiaria coccinea*), a Hawaiian honeycreeper, is territorial when nectar production is moderate but feeds in undefended home ranges when nectar production is either high or low (Carpenter & MacMillen, 1976). In nectarivores, food defense is only cost effective at mid-ranges of nectar production, since when production is high there is a superabundance and no need for defense, and when it is low the cost of defense is higher than the increased food gained (Davies, 1978; Pyke, 1979).

The more economically defensible the food resources, the more likely is the population to be territorially rather than dominance organized. Pronghorn antelope are native to North American grasslands. They nourish a body mass of 50 kg (females) to 56 kg (males) (Mitchell, 1971) by selecting a diet biased toward high quality forbs in the grassland community. In some populations at least some of the time, the more dominant males defend large territories from May through breeding, which occurs in late August or early September. At other times and places males do not defend space, but compete via dominance status to attend one or more females wherever they are. Pronghorn antelope in more productive habitats are territorially organized, but a population in a less productive habitat are dominance organized (Kitchen, 1974; pers. comm.).

Golden winged sunbirds are nectar feeders native to Africa. They are among the largest of a number of sunbird species at around 16 g (Gill & Wolf, 1975). They are closely adapted to feeding on a native flowering plant (*Leonotis nepetifolia*). Where they are the dominant member of their guild the males can establish feeding territories and exclude both conspecifics and other nectar feeders. Nearly all the costs and benefits of territoriality can be expressed in calories, and it is easy to count the calories available in leonotis at any one time and place. Therefore we can readily make and test predictions about the economics of territoriality in this system.

In general, golden winged sunbirds hold territories when the extra nectar in defended flowers is enough to offset the extra costs of defending them (Fig. 2.2). They relax their territorial defense when nectar levels are high and defense no longer increases them enough to offset its costs. For species that defend territories by flying or swimming, wind or water current increases the cost of territorial defense without increasing its benefits. Therefore, all other things being equal, birds in a windier

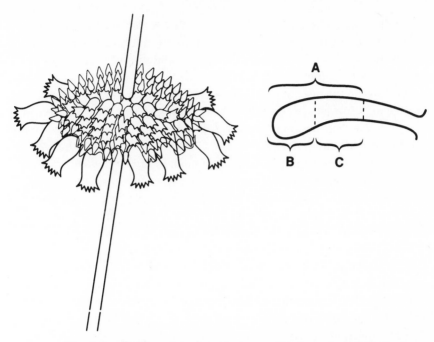

Fig. 2.2. Golden-winged and bronzy sunbirds preferentially feed on *Leonotis nepetifolia*. An inflorescence of this plant is made up of many flowers (left). An individual flower is shown (right). A defended flower has more nectar (A) than an undefended flower (B). The nectar due to territorial defense (C) is the benefit that may justify the costs of territorial defense.

environment or fish in a swift stream should be less likely to be territorial (see also chapter 4).

Differences in predator pressure are sometimes associated with territoriality as an alternative to feeding in an undefended home range. An insular subspecies of the desert woodrat *Neotoma lepida latirostra* is territorial, whereas most desert woodrats are central-place foragers, defending only their nests. Vaughan & Schwartz (1980) suggested this subspecies may be territorial because there is no avian predator on the island to add predation risks to the costs of patrolling and marking.

Diseases and parasites may influence the relative costs and benefits of territory versus an undefended home range. To the extent that territorial behavior reduces the risk of exposure to diseases and parasites carried by conspecifics, it might be favored and hence be more likely in areas of higher incidence of communicable diseases and parasites (Freeland, 1976). Territoriality might also function to manage the level of exposure to the disease, making it possible to approach a degree of exposure which would stimulate the immune system to create antibodies against the disease without enough exposure to have a debilitating case of the disease (B. Hart, pers. comm.).

A change in the distribution of resources other than food can support a change in the social system. When the water in the Mara River in Kenya was high, the distribution of hippos (*Hippopotamus amphibius*) was one territorial male to a pool (Karstad & Hudson, 1986). When the water decreased some of the pools became too small to support a male, and the males in them moved to another pool where they were subordinate to the established male. This change may be a change either to a dominance system or to a dominion system. This case is interesting because the resource that drives the system is not the one males compete for directly. The territorial male can share the water without sharing the females, so the immigrating male can get a critical resource without diluting the resident male's supply of the limiting resource – females.

Ecological determination of this shift may occur more complexly. For example, the response may depend on co-variance of determinants. Pygmy sunfish are territorial when prey are clumped, but they are also territorial when prey are dispersed and the population is of mid-range density (Rubenstein, 1981b).

Species that are organized by territoriality in lower density populations may be organized differently in higher populations. Arizona chuckwallas (*Sauromalus obesus*) are often organized by territoriality. However, a complete failure of most of the plant community in a drought produced an abnormal population density at the remaining concentrations of edible plants. The groups that formed were organized by despotism (Berry, 1974). Perhaps despotism appears facultatively in species that lack a predisposition to shift to dominance relations as an alternative to territoriality.

2.10   DETERMINANTS OF TERRITORIALITY AND FLOCKS OR SCHOOLS AS DETERMINANTS

When food territories are held by food competitors, conspecific or not, individuals often respond by flocking or schooling. Striped parrotfish (*Scarus croicensis*) feed solitarily in undefended home ranges, in territories, or in large schools. The schools often form when prime feeding areas are controlled by territorial competitors. The schools overwhelm or dilute the territorial defense and so apparently function to give their members access to defended food (Ogden & Buckman, 1973; Robertson *et al.*, 1976). Flocking-schooling probably functions to reduce risk when predator pressure is high (Hamilton, 1971), so it is not surprising that increases in predator pressure or predator exposure are correlated with flocking or schooling in species that are territorial in other circumstances. Reedbuck (*Redunca arundinum*) hold territories in dense cover, but when fire or clearing remove their cover and increase predator sight distance they often form small herds (Jungius, 1971). Foraging shorebirds shift from territoriality to flocks when predators appear (Myers *et al.*, 1979a,b). All these instances suggest that the species involved will manifest territoriality when it is economically justified and physically possible but shift to other strategies when either of those conditions does not hold.

3

Intraspecific variation in mating and parental-care system

3.1 MONOGAMY, POLYGYNY, PROMISCUITY, POLYGYNANDRY, SERIAL POLYANDRY, AND SIMULTANEOUS POLYANDRY AS ALTERNATIVE MATING SYSTEMS

These mating systems differ in two ways: (1) the degree to which it is possible to predict which individuals will copulate together from a knowledge of their relationships, and (2) the degree of exclusivity of copulation between particular males and females. The conceptual beginning point of all mating systems is promiscuity. Using promiscuity as a starting point, we may regard all other mating systems as manifesting a reduction in randomness and, working from an adaptationist perspective, a reduction in randomness that contributes an increase in fitness (Fig. 3.1).

In a promiscuous system pairing is random in the sense that the partners in copulation cannot be predicted from a knowledge of the relationships between individual males and females. (Some prediction may be possible from a knowledge of the interactions of males and females with members of their own sex, but that is a different matter.) There appear to be combinations of species and circumstances in which promiscuity is an outcome conferring high fitness. However, most species in most circumstances mate in a way that is to some degree predictable from a knowledge of the relationships between individual males and females. Some species have shown several types of mating systems, but it is more common to see one or the other of a set of two expressed by a particular species.

Idealized monogamy is sharply distinct from randomness. In this system, each male and each female breeds with only one individual. Monogamy is most often reported in birds. However, it is increasingly

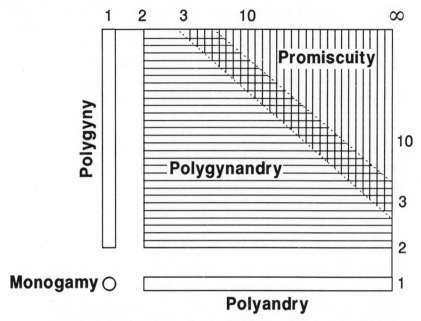

Fig. 3.1. Mating systems can be defined according to the number of individuals each member of each sex mates with. The distinction between polygynandry and promiscuity is necessarily arbitrary and cannot be generally defined.

clear that in many species we have considered to be monogamous, the behavior of some individuals all of the time, and many individuals part of the time, does not conform to this strict definition of monogamy. That is, copulations occur which are not predictable from knowledge of the relationships between individual males and females. Extrapair copulations have been observed in a number of species (e.g., many waterfowl (McKinney *et al.*, 1978), indigo buntings (*Passerina cyanea*) (Westneat, 1987a,b), tree swallows (*Tachycineta bicolor*) (Lombardo, 1986)); in some species mixed parentage of presumably monogamous broods indicates that these copulations are sometimes fertile (Gowaty & Karlin, 1984).

Polygyny also involves reduction in the randomness of promiscuity. In an idealized form each copulating male copulates with more than one female and each copulating female copulates with only one male, and we can predict all partners by knowing their relationships. However, in practice the reduction of randomness from promiscuity is not always as complete as that definition implies, as females may copulate with other males (Gowaty & Karlin, 1984).

The current working distinctions between promiscuity and all forms of polyandry are clear when expressed as platonic ideals. In serial polyandry the female mates with more than one male during a season but only mates with the second after she has ceased to mate with the first. In simultaneous polyandry the female bonds with several males during the same part of the same season. Simultaneous polyandry requires that the female accept at least two, possibly more, courting males. Cooperative polyandry, in which several males attend a single female and clutch at a single nest, requires greater male–male tolerance than does promiscuity. Some instances of more than one of these alternatives being observed in a single species are reported in Tables 3.1 to 3.7.

3.2   MATING SYSTEMS BACKGROUND

Vertebrate mating systems are always shaped by at least two forces: the ecological and demographic setting to which the mates must adjust, and the mix of conflict and concordance in and between the interests of the mates themselves. The many organismic and environmental variables thus brought into play create rich and intricate puzzles that have challenged and intrigued behavioral biologists from Darwin to the present. Mating systems were a major feature of every general treatment of socioecology in the early to mid-1960s (e.g., Eisenberg, 1962; Crook, 1965) and continue to the present (e.g., Wrangham, 1986; Davies, 1989; Clutton-Brock, 1990).

Most essays and reviews on the evolution of mating systems have emphasized ecological variables as determinants. Emlen & Oring (1977) wrote a compelling interpretation of mating systems from this perspective. But the conflict of interest between the mates is increasingly seen as an important determinant. Trivers (1972) has stated this conflict and its implications clearly. Maynard Smith (1978, 1982) has shown that these conflicts are nicely modeled by game theory. They are increasingly incorporated into mating system theory (e.g., Davies, 1989).

This history, and the interplay of these trends, are illustrated by some highlights of the development of the polygyny threshold as an explanatory concept. Verner (1964) argued that each territorial male bird will have finite resources in his territory. Resources up to a certain level will support a single nesting female and her offspring. Such a territory will probably have a monogamous pair breeding there. But if the male's territory holds enough additional resources to support two breeding females, the opportunities in this territory, when weighed against those

Table 3.1. *Monogamy and polygyny as alternative social systems.*

Species	Differences in circumstances (M – when monogamous, P – when polygynous, NKD signifies no known difference in circumstances)	References
Slimy sculpin *Cottus cognatus*	More P where nest sites limited	Mousseau & Collins, 1987
Red sea damselfish *Dascyllus marginatus*	P when male hold coral head large enough for more than one female	Fricke, 1980
Cichlid *Cichlasoma panamense*	More P when fewer predators, more females	Townshend & Wootton, 1985
Cichlid *Cichlasoma nigrofasciatum*	P when sex ratio female biased, size differences small	Keenleyside, 1985
Cichlid *Lamprologus brichardi*	NKD; P when male intruder pressure not too high	Taborsky & Limberger, 1981; Limberger, 1983
Tree lizard *Liolaemus tenuis*	P when male 'holds' tree large enough for more than one female	Manzur & Fuentes, 1979
Tree lizard *Urosaurus ornatus*	More P in larger trees	M'Closkey *et al.*, 1987
Shag *Phalacrocaras aristotelis*	NKD	Potts, 1968
Mute swan *Cygnus olor*	NKD	Dewar, 1937
Black swan *Cygnus atratus*	P in captivity	Braithwaite, 1981
Magpie goose *Anseranas semipalmata*	NKD	Frith & Davies, 1961
Bar-headed goose *Anser indicus*	P in captivity, female biased sex ratio	Lamprecht, 1987; Lamprecht & Buhrow, 1987
Canada goose *Branta canadensis*	NKD; P when trio familiar	Kossack, 1950; Fabricius & Boyd, 1985
Canada goose *Branta canadensis maxima*	P when few males available	Brakhage, 1965
African comb duck *Sarkidiornis melanotos*	P when sufficient resources available for females to settle	Siegfried, 1978

Table 3.1.   (*cont.*)

Species	Differences in circumstances (M – when monogamous, P – when polygynous, NKD signifies no known difference in circumstances)	References
Bufflehead *Bucephala albeola*	P when widowed females available	Gauthier, 1986
Barrow's goldeneye *Bucephala islandica*	P attributed to philopatry, widowing, familiarity	Savard, 1986
Pochard *Aythya ferina*	NKD	Rolls, 1983
Red grouse *Lagopus lagopus scoticus*	More P when more food in territory	Miller & Watson, 1978
Willow ptarmigan *Lagopus lagopus*	P when sex ratio female biased	Hannon, 1983, 1984; Martin, 1984, 1989
Moorhen *Gallinula chloropus*	More P when females related	Gibbons, 1986
Temminck's stint *Calidris temminckii*	NKD	Hilden, 1975
Herring gull *Larus argentatus*	NKD	Shugart & Southern, 1977; Shugart, 1980; Fitch & Shugart, 1983
Ring-billed gull *Larus delawarensis*	NKD; P when sex ratio female biased	Conover *et al.*, 1979; Kovacs & Ryder, 1983; LaGrenade & Mousseau, 1983
Black-headed gull *Larus ridibundus*	More P in captivity	van Rhijn & Groothuis, 1985
Mountain plover *Charadrius montanus*	P when food supply erratic	Graul, 1973
Snowy owl *Nyctea scandiaca*	NKD	Watson, 1957
Barn owl *Tyto alba*	NKD	Marti, 1987
Hawk owl *Surnia ulula*	NKD	Sonerud *et al.*, 1987
Tengmalm's owl *Aegolius funereus*	More P when food more abundant	Carlsson *et al.*, 1987
Northern saw-whet owl *Aegolius acadicus*	More P when food and nest sites concentrated	Marks *et al.*, 1987

Table 3.1.   (*cont.*)

Species	Differences in circumstances (M – when monogamous, P – when polygynous, NKD signifies no known difference in circumstances)	References
Marsh harrier *Circus aerguinosus*	NKD	Altenburg *et al.*, 1982
European hen harrier (Northern harrier) *Circus cyaneus*	NKD; more P among older males; more P when more food; more P among males displaying more; more P among males displaying provisioning performance better	Jourdain, 1926b; Balfour & Cadbury, 1979; Picozzi, 1983, 1984; Hamerstrom *et al.*, 1985; Simmons *et al.*, 1986, 1987; Simmons, 1988a,b
Snail kite *Rostrhamus sociabilis*	P when food abundant	Beissinger, 1986
Peregrine *Falco peregrinus*	NKD	Walker, 1987
Sparrow hawk *Accipiter nisus*	NKD	Greeves, 1926; Jourdain, 1926a
Kestrel *Falco tinnunculus tinnunculus*	NKD	Jourdain, 1926a
Groove-billed ani *Crotophaga sulcirostris*	Occasionally P when monogamous pairs breed	Vehrencamp, 1978
Pied flycatcher *Ficedula hypoleuca*	P when male deceives female, when territory better; older males more polygynous; M when few late arriving females; more P in more dense population; NKD	von Haartman, 1951; Alatalo & Lundberg, 1984; Nyholm, 1984; Virolainen, 1984; Harvey *et al.*, 1985; Alatalo *et al.*, 1986
Acadian flycatcher *Empidonax virescens*	NKD	Mumford, 1964
Willow flycatcher *Empidonax traillii*	NKD	Prescott, 1986
Least flycatcher *Empidonax minimus*	NKD	Briskie & Sealy, 1987
Western wood pewee *Contopus sordidulus*	NKD	Eckhardt, 1976

Table 3.1.   (*cont.*)

Species	Differences in circumstances (M – when monogamous, P – when polygynous, NKD signifies no known difference in circumstances)	References
Purple martin *Progne subis*	NKD; Early males more P	Southern, 1959; Brown, 1975; 1979
Barn swallow *Hirundo rustica*	NKD	Richardson, 1957
Red-breasted swallow *Hirundo semirufa*	P with inexperienced secondary female	Earle, 1987
Bank swallow *Riparia riparia*	NKD	Stoner, 1939
Tree swallow *Iridoprocne bicolor*	More P when sex ratio female biased; P when food abundant & nest sites limited	Shelley, 1935; Quinney, 1983
Rook *Corvus frugilegus*	P when more females	Green, 1982
Jackdaw *Corvus monedula*	P follows incomplete supplanting of mated female by unmated male	Roell, 1979
Florida scrub jay *Aphelocoma coerulescens coerulescens*	NKD	Woolfenden, 1976
Magpie *Pica pica*	NKD	Birkhead *et al.*, 1985
European starling *Sturnus vulgaris*	P when few nest sites	Stouffer *et al.*, 1988
Northern shrike *Lanius excubitor*	NKD	Yosef & Pinshow, 1988
Blue tit *Parus caerulus*	More P in better, more productive habitat	Dhondt, 1987a,b
Black-capped chickadee *Parus atricapillus*	NKD	Smith, 1967
Nuthatch *Sitta europaea*	P when widowed territory neighbor joins pair	Matthysen, 1986
Treecreeper *Certhia familiaris*	P when neighboring female widowed	Harper, 1986
Short-billed marsh wren *Cistothorus elatensis*	More P when nesting in *Scirpus fluvitalis*	Crawford, 1977
Marsh wren *Cistothorus palustris*	More P in western population with longer breeding season	Kroodsma & Canady, 1985
Long-billed marsh wren *Telmatodytes palustris*	More P when habitat more saturated	Verner, 1964

Table 3.1.   (*cont.*)

Species	Differences in circumstances (M – when monogamous, P – when polygynous, NKD signifies no known difference in circumstances)	References
House wren *Troglodytes aedon*	More territorial males more P?; Possibly more P when territorial neighbor ill	Kendeigh, 1941; Freed, 1986a,b
Dipper *Cinclus mexicanus*	P in larger territories lacking neighbors at one boundary	Price & Bock, 1973
Eastern bluebird *Sialia sialis*	NKD	Gowaty, 1983
Mockingbird *Mimus polyglottos*	P when territorial neighbor leaves; NKD	Logan & Rulli, 1981; Breitwisch *et al.*, 1986
Black-throated blue warbler *Dendroica caerulescens*	NKD	Petit *et al.*, 1988
Fan-tailed warbler *Cisticola juncidis*	P in rice fields	Avery, 1982
Marsh warbler *Acrocephalus palustris*	NKD	Dowset-Lemaire, 1979
Willow warbler *Phylloscopus trochilus*	P when neighbor's territory abandoned	Lawn, 1978
Wood warbler *Phylloscopus sibilatrix*	More P when nesting territories limited; NKD	Temrin, 1989; Temrin & Jakobsson, 1988
Yellow warbler *Dendroica petechia*	P in larger territories, P possibly due to cowbird disturbance; NKD	DellaSala, 1985, 1986; Reid & Sealy, 1986
Prairie warbler *Dendroica discolor*	NKD	Nolan, 1963
Kirtland's warbler *Dendroica kirtlandii*	More P when habitat more saturated	Radabaugh, 1972
Fan-tailed warbler *Cisticola juncidis*	NKD	Ueda, 1984
Common yellowthroat *Geothlypis trichas*	P when sex ratio female biased	Powell & Jones, 1978
Isabelline chat *Oenanthe isabellina*	More P in longer season?	Ivanitsky, 1978
Dunnock *Prunella modularis*	More P when food more patchy	Davies & Lundberg, 1984

Table 3.1.   (*cont.*)

Species	Differences in circumstances (M – when monogamous, P – when polygynous, NKD signifies no known difference in circumstances)	References
Indigo bunting *Passerina cyanea*	Older males more P; NKD	Carey & Nolan, 1975, 1979; Westneat, 1988b
Lark bunting *Calamospiza melanocorys*	P in territory with more shade	Pleszczynska, 1978
Heuglin's masked weaver *Ploceus heuglini*	P when colonial	Grimes, 1973
Dickcissel *Spiza americana*	More P where one male controls more nest sites	Zimmerman, 1966
Ipswich sparrow	P at low population densities	Stobo & McLaren, 1975
Savanna sparrow *Passerculus sandwichensis*	M in short breeding season latitude; P elsewhere, M at Queen's University Tundra Biology Station; more M at higher latitudes	Welsh, 1975; Weatherhead, 1979a,b; Rising, 1987a,b
Chipping sparrow *Spizella passerina passerina*	NKD	Walkinshaw, 1959
White-crowned sparrow *Zonotricia leucophrys*	More P when habitat saturated; more P when testosterone implanted	Petrinovich & Patterson, 1978; Wingfield, 1984
Song sparrow *Melospiza melodia*	P when excess females; P when testosterone implanted	Nice, 1937; Smith *et al.*, 1982; Wingfield, 1984
Swamp sparrow *Melospiza georgiana*	NKD	Willson, 1966
Western lark sparrow *Chondestes grammacus strigatus*	NKD	Knowles, 1938
Lapwing *Vanellus vanellus*	NKD	Wilson, 1967
Bobolink *Dolichonyx oryzivorus*	P when females locally abundant	Wootton *et al.*, 1986
Common grackle *Quiscalus quiscala*	NKD	Howe, 1979

Table 3.1. (*cont.*)

Species	Differences in circumstances (M – when monogamous, P – when polygynous, NKD signifies no known difference in circumstances)	References
Brown-headed cowbird *Molothrus ater*	More M when population less dense; P when many host nests & sex ratio female biased; NKD	Duffy, 1982; Teather & Robertson, 1986; Yokel, 1986
Blackbird *Agelaius* spp.	P where have widespread feeding areas but restricted nest sites	Orians, 1961
House finch *Carpodacus mexicanus frontalis*	NKD	Michener, 1925
Zebra finch *Poephila guttata*	NKD	Burley, 1986
Beaver *Castor canadensis*	P when population more dense	Busher *et al.*, 1983
Bushy-tailed woodrat *Neotoma cinerea*	M on small rock outcrop, P on larger rock outcrop	Escherick, 1981
Prairie vole *Microtus ochrogaster*	More P in winter	Getz *et al.*, 1987
Yellow-bellied marmot *Marmota flaviventris*	M when dominant female socially intolerant	Armitage & Downhower, 1974; Johns & Armitage, 1979
European rabbit *Oryctolagus cuniculus*	P when females grouped; M when soil precludes large warrens	Cowan & Bell, 1986; Roberts, 1987
Pika *Ochotona princeps*	More P when population density low	Smith & Ivins, 1984
Weddell seal *Leptonychotes weddelli*	Dispersal with cracks in ice pack; at many cracks, some M, rest P	Jouventin & Cornet, 1980
Hawaiian monk seal *Monachus schauinslandi*	P when females concentrated, M when dispersed	Jouventin & Cornet, 1980
Hooded seal *Cystophora cristata*	P when females clustered?	Boness *et al.*, 1988
Red fox *Vulpes vulpes*	P when sex ratio female biased? P when more food in male territory	MacDonald, 1979, 1980, 1981; von Schantz, 1981

Table 3.1.   (*cont.*)

Species	Differences in circumstances (M – when monogamous, P – when polygynous, NKD signifies no known difference in circumstances)	References
White-tailed deer *Odocoileus virginianus*	P in more open habitat, females in larger social groups	Hirth, 1977
Feral horse *Equus caballus*	NKD	Miller, 1981
Saddle-backed tamarin *Saguinus fuscicollis*	NKD	Terborgh & Goldizen, 1985; Goldizen, 1988
Pileated gibbon *Hylobates pileatus*	NKD	Srikosamatara & Brockelman, 1987
Sunda Island leaf monkey *Presbytis aygula*	NKD	Ruhiyat, 1983
Mentawai snub-nosed langur *Simias concolor*	More P where population density higher	Watanabe, 1981

elsewhere, may induce a second female to settle there. Such a territory is above the 'polygyny threshold'.

Verner & Willson (1966) surveyed the literature on avian breeding systems and concluded that those species breeding in habitats where territories were likely to exceed the polygyny threshold tended to be 'polygynous species'. Orians (1969) advanced the thinking on avian polygyny by specifying more exactly the ecological and demographic conditions that would cross the polygyny threshold. He also developed the relationship between these variables more clearly. These theoretical developments stimulated a great deal of empirical research, which generally has been seen as supporting this threshold model.

However, Davies (1989) argued that this literature has neglected the central position of conflicts of interest between the mates in determining the breeding system. He argued that ecology simply constrains the possible social system outcomes the interacting birds may produce, and it is only indirectly a determinant of that outcome. He suggested that what has evolved is not so much adaptation to the ecology but behavioral

Table 3.2. *Monogamy and promiscuity as alternative social systems.*

Species	Differences in circumstances (M – when monogamous, PR – when promiscuous, NKD signifies no known difference in circumstances)	References
Red sea damselfish *Dascyllus marginatus*	PR when coral heads large enough for more than one male territory	Fricke, 1980
Pukeko *Porphyrio porphyrio melanotus*	NKD	Craig, 1979
Shag *Phalacrocarax aristotelis*	NKD	Harris, 1982
White ibis *Endocimus albus*	NKD	Kushlan, 1973
Temminck's stint *Calidris temminckii*	NKD	Hilden, 1975
Western gull *Larus occidentalis*	PR possibly associated with unbalanced sex ratio (more females), P when more food	Hunt & Hunt, 1977; Pierrotti, 1981
Ring-billed gull *Larus delawarensis*	PR possibly associated with unbalanced sex ratio (more females)	Conover *et al.*, 1979
California gull *Larus californicus*	PR possibly associated with unbalanced sex ratio (more females)	Conover *et al.*, 1979
Brown-headed cowbird *Molothrus ater*	PR when few host nests available; More M among larger, dominant males	Elliott, 1980; Ankney & Scott, 1982
Brown hyena *Hyaena brunnea*	PR when territories support 2+ breeding females	Mills, 1982
European rabbit *Oryctolagus cuniculus*	More PR when females grouped	Cowan & Bell, 1986

strategies pursued by each individual which are constrained by, or adjusted to, the ecological setting.

These perspectives are not really contradictory; in many cases advocates of each would probably make the same predictions. However, they have quite different emphases and reflect differences in world view that will influence research. For example, if one were to initiate an analysis of the assessment mechanisms breeding birds use, a follower of the

Table 3.3.   *Monogamy and polygynandry as alternative social systems.*

Species	Differences in circumstances (M – when monogamous, PO – when polygynandrous, NKD signifies no known difference in circumstances)	References
Dusky moorhen *Gallinula tenebrosa*	NKD	Garnett, 1978, 1980
Acorn woodpecker *Melanerpes formicivorus*	M when no acorn storage trees, migrate; PO when stored mast abundant	Stacey & Bock, 1978; Stacey, 1979a; Stacey & Koenig, 1984
Dunnock *Prunella modularis*	More PO when food more patchy	Davies & Lundberg, 1984

Table 3.4.   *Polygyny and promiscuity as alternative social systems.*

Species	Differences in circumstances (PO – when polygynous, PR – when promiscuous, NKD signifies no known difference in circumstances)	References
Dusky moorhen *Galinula tenebrosa*	NKD	Garnett, 1980
Temminck's stint *Calidris temminckii*	NKD	Hilden, 1975
Ani *Crotophaga* spp.	NKD	Davis, 1941
Salt marsh harvest mouse *Reithrodontomys raviventris*	NKD	Fisler, 1965
Deer mouse *Peromyscus maniculatus*	PO at high population density	Mihok, 1979
European rabbit *Oryctolagus cuniculus*	PO when females grouped	Cowan & Bell, 1986

Table 3.5. *Polygyny and polygynandry as alternative social systems.*

Species	Differences in circumstances (PO – when polygynous, PA – when polygynandrous, NKD signifies no known difference in circumstances)	References
Feral horse *Equus caballus*	PO in one male bands; PA in multiple male bands	Miller, 1981
Red colobus *Colobus badius*	More PA when multimale group hierarchy unstable	Struhsaker & Leland, 1979
Mangabey *Cercocebus albigena*	More PA when multimale group hierarchy unstable	Struhsaker & Leland, 1979
Redtail monkey *Cercopithecus ascanius*	NKD	Cords, 1984
Gorilla *Gorilla gorilla*	NKD	Harcourt *et al.*, 1980

ecological emphasis would tend to look for assessment of ecological features such as the distribution and abundance of food, cover, free water, etc. In contrast, a follower of the game theoretic approach might look for assessment of social strategies that individuals in the same subpopulation are following.

3.3   ECOLOGICAL DETERMINANTS OF MATING SYSTEMS VARIATION

Ecological circumstances correlate strongly with mating systems (Emlen & Oring, 1977; Wittenberger, 1981; Oring, 1982; Clutton-Brock, 1990). In the context of this chapter, it will be useful to ask what circumstances favor a shift from (or toward) randomness in the directions of monogamy or polygyny.

3.3.1   Patch size

In several cases the alternative mating patterns seem to be a consequence of the size of the available resource patch. A species of damselfish, *Dascyllus aruanus*, takes shelter in small openings among coral-reef heads. The active colony of coral polyps that produce a growing coral head are economically defendable and the heads create a patchy distri-

Table 3.6. *Monogamy and serial polyandry as alternative social systems.*

Species	Differences in circumstances (M – when monogamous, P – when polyandrous, NKD signifies no known difference in circumstances)	References
Snowy plover *Charadrius alexandrinus*	NKD; More P when sex ratio male biased	Lessells, 1984; Warriner *et al.*, 1986
Mountain plover *Charadrius montanus*	P when food erratic	Graul, 1973
Killdeer *Charadrius vociferus*	NKD	Brunton, 1988
Spotted sandpiper *Actitis macularia*	P where sex ratio male biased; more P when higher density	Oring & Knudson, 1972; Maxson & Oring, 1980
Sanderling *Calidris alba*	P in good breeding conditions	Parmelee & Payne, 1973
Dunlin *Calidris alpina*	P in good breeding conditions	Soikkeli, 1967
Temminck's stint *Calidris temminckii*	NKD	Hilden, 1975
Red phalarope *Phalaropus fulicarius*	More P when longer breeding season; P when sex ratio male biased	Schamel & Tracy, 1977; Reynolds, 1985
Red-necked phalarope *Phalaropus lobatus*	P when sex ratio male biased	Reynolds, 1985, 1987
Wilson's phalarope *Phalaropus tricolor*	NKD; P when more males available	Colwell, 1986; Colwell & Oring, 1988
Snail kite *Rostrhamus sociabilis*	P when food abundant	Beissinger, 1986
California valley quail *Callipepla californica*	More P when more food	Leopold, 1977
Bank swallow (Sand martin) *Riparia riparia*	NKD; more P in older birds after first brood failure	Stoner, 1939; Cowley, 1983
Marsh warbler *Acrocephalus palustris*	NKD	Dowsett-Lemaire, 1979
Kirtland's warbler *Dendroica kirtlandii*	NKD	Radabaugh, 1972
Bay-winged cowbird *Molothrus badius*	NKD	Fraga, 1972

Table 3.7.   *Monogamy and simultaneous polyandry as alternative social systems.*

Species	Differences in circumstances (M – when monogamous, P – when polyandrous, NKD signifies no known difference in circumstances)	References
Harris' hawk *Parabuteo unicinctus*	NKD; NKD, P not conclusively demonstrated	Mader, 1975a,b, 1977, 1979; Bednarz, 1987
Galapagos hawk *Buteo galapagoensis*	M pairs remnants of P groups	Faaborg, 1986
Tasmanian native hen *Tribonyx mortierii*	NKD	Ridpath, 1972
Dusky moorhen *Gallinula tenebrosa*	NKD	Garnett, 1980
Dwarf cuckoo *Coccyzus pumilus*	NKD	Ralph, 1975
Pied flycatcher *Muscicapa hypoleuca*	NKD	von Haartman, 1951
Nuthatch *Sitta europaea*	P when widowered territory neighbor joins pair	Matthysen, 1986
Superb blue wren *Malurus cyaneus*	NKD	Rowley, 1965
Northern mockingbird *Mimus polyglottos*	NKD	Fulk *et al.*, 1987
Eastern bluebird *Sialia sialis sialis*	NKD	Laskey, 1947
Oven-bird *Seiurus aurocapillus*	NKD	Hann, 1940
Dunnock *Prunella modularis*	More P when food more patchy	Davies & Lundberg, 1984
Zebra finch *Poephila guttata*	NKD	Burley, 1986
Saddle-backed tamarin *Saguinus fuscicollis*	NKD; P when no helpers in group	Terborgh & Goldizen, 1985; Goldizen, 1987, 1988
Prairie vole *Microtus ochrogaster*	More P in winter	Getz *et al.*, 1987
Beaver *Castor canadensis*	Possibly P when population dense	Busher *et al.*, 1983

bution of that resource. A male defends an area large enough in which to live and breed, and he will breed with all the females that enter it. Female home ranges extend over an entire coral head, but not beyond it. They breed with all the males they encounter in their home range. The whole of a small coral head is defended by an individual male. If such a coral head is large enough for only one female the mating system is monogamy. If it is large enough for two or three females the mating system is polygyny. Two or more males divide larger coral heads into territories and several females establish home ranges that cover the entire coral head. Such a set of damselfish breeds polygynandrously (Fricke, 1977) (Fig. 3.2). Small rocky outcrops accommodate a territorial male bushy-tailed woodrat (*Neotoma floridana*) and one female, which breed monogamously (Escherick, 1981). Small trees accommodate a territorial male tree lizard (*Anolis aeneus*) and one female, also breeding monogamously (Manzur & Fuentes, 1979). Larger trees or outcrops have a territorial male and more than one female which breed polygynously.

3.3.2   Patch quality

Variation in resource patch quality is also associated with alternative mating systems. Male red foxes (*Vulpes vulpes*) tend to defend areas of relatively constant size. Most such territories contain one female, and the pair are monogamous. But the amount of food within territories can vary considerably. Moehlman (1989) predicted that red fox mating systems will alternate between polygyny and monogamy depending upon the richness of resource patches. Her prediction is supported strongly by Zabel & Taggart (1989), and to a lesser extent by von Schantz (1981) and MacDonald (1981).

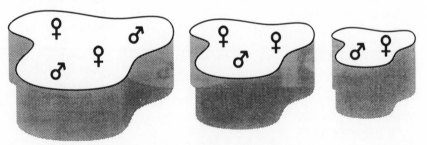

Fig. 3.2.   Mating system determined by size of habitat patch. As patch size increases the mating system changes from monogamy to polygyny (e.g., Red Sea damselfish, tree lizards, and bushy-tailed woodrats). Still larger patches produced polygynandry in Red Sea damselfish.

Zabel & Taggart (1989) observed red foxes that fed primarily on nesting seabirds. In years when seabirds were abundant, most females bred in a polygynous set, where they had the same reproductive success as monogamous females in the same population. Some dens had helpers. When the seabirds failed to reproduce (after an El Nino), all the reproductive groups became monogamous and there were fewer helpers. (An El Nino is a warming of the surface of the Pacific Ocean off Peru that causes fish production to decline for a season.)

There is at least one example of monogamy alternating with polygyny that is apparently produced by a random process. The mating system of male bobolinks (*Dolichonyx oryzivorus*) holding territories in a uniform habitat was determined by whether one or more than one female happened to settle in their territory (Wootton *et al.*, 1986) (Fig. 3.3).

Variation in potential food storage appears to act as a determinant of the breeding system of acorn woodpeckers (*Melanerpes formicivorus*). A group may store up to 10,000 acorns in holes drilled into dead trees or the bark of living pines (MacRoberts & MacRoberts, 1976; Stacey & Ligon, 1987). These stored acorns nourish them through the winter. In areas with suitable storage trees they are year-round residents, living in groups of up to ten adults breeding polyandrously, polygynously or polygynandrously (Fig. 3.4). Where there are few storage trees, they often breed as monogamous pairs (Stacey & Bock, 1978; Stacey & Ligon, 1987). However, one population has been described as breeding communally without storage facilities (Kattan, 1988) (see also chapter 4).

3.3.3   Competition, population and sex ratios

Intensity of competition for a resource may vary with the form of breeding system. When competition is high a male may be able to control only enough of a limiting resource to support one female. If he could control enough resources for two females he might increase his success by breeding polygynously (Orians, 1969; Verner & Willson, 1966). This is illustrated by a population of dippers (*Cinclus mexicanus*) breeding in linear territories along a riparian habitat. Boundaries were defended only where there was an adjoining territory. Most of the males within the linear series had one female and defended two boundaries. The territories at each end of the series had only one defended boundary, were larger, and had two females (Price & Bock, 1973).

Increased total abundance of voles produced an increase in the percentage of polygyny in a population of northern harriers and a year to year shift from monogamy to polygyny in individual males (Simmons *et*

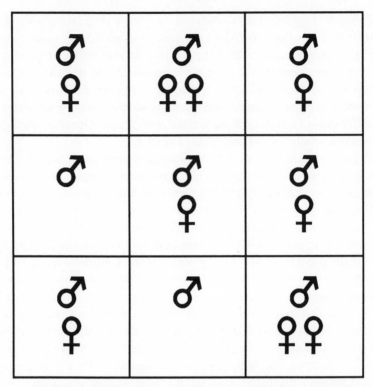

Fig. 3.3. Mating system variation in bobolinks in a homogeneous habitat. The variation is the result of females settling randomly (Wootton *et al.*, 1986). If resources are abundant and not patchy, the habitat can be equally partitioned by territory holders. Random settling by mates could produce variation among the alternative systems of monogamy, polygyny and polyandry that was not systematically related to ecological variation (demonstrated to be the source of polygyny and monogamy as alternative systems in bobolinks (Wootton *et al.*, 1986)).

al., 1986). Northern harriers are marsh-nesting raptors that feed largely on small rodents. They are widespread in both North America and Europe. (Until recently the European and North American populations were classified as separate species.) Some nest polygynously and others monogamously throughout their range. Polygyny is more frequent on Orkney Island and has been attributed to a skewed sex ratio (Balfour & Cadbury, 1979; Picozzi, 1984). Polygyny varied from 11 to 40% of nests in a single Canadian population. There was a strong positive correlation between the population of voles (*Microtus pennsylvanicus*) and the percentage of polygynous nests over five years (Simmons *et al.*, 1986) (Fig. 3.5).

Sex ratios may constrain or increase the options available. If females become relatively more abundant the mating system may move toward polygyny. For example, experimental removal of male willow ptarmigan (*Lagopus lagopus*) increased the incidence of polygyny in a territorial system (Hannon, 1983, 1984; Martin, 1989). Particular diseases or patterns of predation may increase the number of males per female in a population or vice versa. Human persecution may produce a shift in sex ratio in species in which one sex is more vulnerable, or more sought after, than the other. Perhaps this is the reason why Kleiman (1977) predicts polygyny in coyote populations experiencing high levels of human persecution. (This assumes that human persecution is more likely to take males than females.)

3.3.4   Wind speed

Wind speed may also influence the mating systems of flying animals. Wind increases the time and energy spent during round trips. Forms of breeding that are already only marginally cost-effective might become

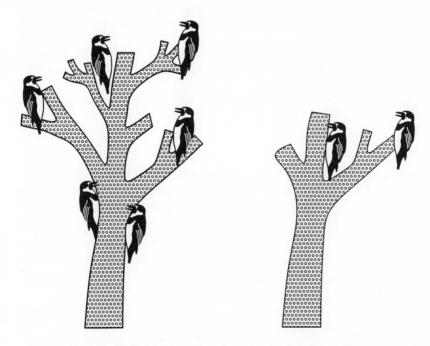

Fig. 3.4. Loss of acorn storage reduced the size of a social group of acorn woodpeckers and changed the social system from helpers at the nest to parents-only care (data from Stacey & Ligon, 1987).

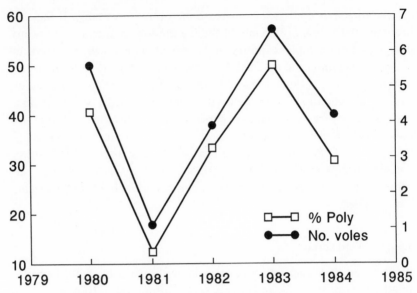

Fig. 3.5. Percentage of female northern harriers breeding polygynously (left vertical axis) plotted against the number of voles caught per 100 trap nights in August (right vertical axis). The vole population in May did not correlate as strongly with the percentage of females breeding polygynously. The August data are presented because the May vole population was estimated rather than sampled in some of the study years, but it was sampled every year in August (data from Simmons *et al.*, 1986).

cost-ineffective with the increased time and energy. For example, poly-territorial polygyny in the pied flycatcher involves long flights between separate breeding territories. This species varies between monogamy and polyterritorial polygyny (Nyholm, 1984; Harvey *et al.*, 1985). It would be useful to learn if this variation is correlated with differences in wind speed. Wind speed would increase the costs of territoriality in general. As the cost of territoriality increased, the net benefits of resource defense polygyny would decrease.

Ecological determinants of these social systems have been discussed separately, but they are more likely to act in combination. Vectors acting at the same time may act with or contrary to one another. Consequently, predicting will be complicated. Precise predictions will require quantitative descriptions of the force of the vectors.

3.4 ECOLOGICAL DETERMINANTS OF POLYANDRY

Observations of facultative serial polyandry suggest it is a response to unusually favorable circumstances. Populations of California quail (*Callipepla californica*) living in relatively xeric environments manifest serial polyandry in years when food is abundant (Leopold, 1977; Mastrup, in prep.). An unusually long breeding season in a short-season environment can have the same effect. Red phalarope (*Phalaropus fulicaria*) females with a longer breeding season available, either because of yearly variation in their Arctic breeding grounds or because of early arrival at the breeding ground, are likely to abandon their incubating males and mate again (Schamel & Tracy, 1977). In both of these cases facultative serial polyandry enhances female reproduction by making it possible for her to bring off more than one clutch when resources are unusually high. These observations of facultative serial polyandry suggest it is an opportunistic exploitation of unusually rich circumstances.

In contrast, facultative cooperative simultaneous polyandry seems more likely to be a product of environmental limitation. Harris' hawks live in a xeric environment with very low prey density. Trios composed of two males and one female are common, and they may be engaged in cooperative polyandry (Mader, 1975b; but see Bednarz, 1987). Trios fledge 33% more young per nesting attempt than pairs. Thus mated females do better in a polyandrous system. Males do not do as well unless the trio double clutches, as a few trios do (Mader, 1975b). Since females are dominant, they may be able to control suitable breeding areas well enough to present males with the choice of breeding polyandrously or not at all.

Dunnocks are small (14 cm), drab birds that eat seeds and insects. They produce two to three broods per year from nests in deep cover all over Britain and are widespread in Europe. They mate in several different systems, even within a single population, and some individuals change systems from brood to brood. Monogamy, cooperative polyandry and polygyny are all fairly common in nature. Polygynandry is not common, but occurs (Davies & Lundberg, 1984). It appears that each member of each sex pursues the same strategy. The application of these two strategies in a variety of circumstances produces a variety of mating system outcomes.

Females establish home ranges with a certain minimum amount of food and exclude other females from that range. Males establish a range with the maximum number of females they can defend and try to exclude all other males. Where food is sparse the home ranges of females are larger than the territory of one male, and the two or more males that have territories in her home range gradually give up trying to exclude each other and defend the whole space jointly. One male becomes dominant and tries to prevent the subordinate(s) from breeding, while the female encourages them. If the subordinate(s) also breed the group is polyandrous.

If food density is mid-range the female's home range is small enough for one male to defend and the pair breed monogamously. If food patches are abundant female home ranges are smaller still and the territory of one male may encompass two female home ranges. If he cannot exclude all other males another may establish himself there and jointly defend the female home ranges. Both males will breed with all the females, and the result is polygynandry.

Polyandry is rarely observed in mammals, but there are two species in which it has been documented. Saddle-backed tamarins (*Saguinus fuscicollus*) express simultaneous cooperative polyandry, with all males copulating with the female and sharing in the care of the infants (Goldizen, 1987). Although their rain forest environment has high primary productivity, the tamarins must compete for fruit and nectar with more dominant species of primates and more mobile species of birds, so the resources available to the tamarins are sparse (Terborgh & Goldizen, 1985). Consequently a large area must be vigorously defended against conspecifics and additional parental care may be at a premium, making it adaptive for males to accept partners as a way to extend their lives and decrease the mortality of the infants. This is similar to the situation for the Harris hawks, and the polyandrous system may be developed in response to the same variables.

Demographics alone seem able to determine whether monogamy or cooperative simultaneous polyandry will be expressed by naked mole rats (*Heterocephalus glaber*) (Sherman, pers. comm.). In this semi-eusocial mammal there is always only one female in a breeding system. As the males reach a certain size they begin to breed with her (and also to care for young). When there is only one male of that size the system expressed is monogamy, but when there is more than one it is polyandry. Since the males are likely to be closely related, inclusive fitness will help to keep the costs of polyandry low and the benefits high.

3.5   TWO-PARENT, ONE-PARENT, BROOD SPLIT, COMMUNAL CARE, AND HELPERS AT THE NEST AS CARE-GIVING ALTERNATIVES

In a parents-only system the young are cared for by their biological parents and only by them. In a two-parent system both parents give care to all of their joint young. In a one-parent system one parent gives care to all the young and the other gives none. In a brood-split system each parent cares only for certain of the young. In communal care, parents care for their own young and also those of other parents. Helpers at the nest care only for young that are not theirs.

Behaviorally, then, in a two-parent system both parents are responsive to all the young, in a one-parent system only one parent is responsive to any of the young, and in a brood-split system each parent is responsive to some, but not all, of the young. Relationships in communal systems differ from those in parental systems in several ways. Parents in communal systems do not discriminate among the young they are exposed to, while parents in parental systems do. Moreover, many communal systems require increased tolerance between parental adults, which in a parental system would not let a conspecific approach their nest or young. Some instances of more than one of these care-giving alternatives being observed in a single species are reported in Tables 3.8 to 3.11.

3.6   PARENTAL CARE BACKGROUND

Parental care involves a number of costs. Predation risks are often higher, energy may be spent gathering and delivering food, and mobility may be limited by the young's degree of development. When non-parents care for immatures of their own species, i.e., act as helpers, they may bear the additional cost of foregoing reproduction themselves.

One theoretical challenge, then, is to identify the benefits that compensate for these costs. When the good of the species was seen as an appropriate goal of behavior, that was easy. But when the logic of natural selection was applied more rigorously to care-giving behavior the challenge became greater.

The parents themselves clearly benefit by increased fitness: their offspring carry their genes into the next generation. Hamilton's (1964a,b) contribution of kinship selection made it possible to recognize a potential fitness benefit to related care-givers through transmission of shared genes. This offers a rigorous interpretation of helpers at the nest.

However, an alternative explanation of helpers at the nest is that young

Table 3.8.   *Communal care as an alternative to parental care.*

Species	Differences in circumstances (CC – when communal care, PC – when parental care, NKD signifies no known difference in circumstances	References
Magpie goose *Anseranas semipalmata*	NKD	Frith & Davies, 1961
Eider *Somateria mollissima*	CC when gull predation high	Ahlen & Andersson, 1970
Moorhen *Gallinula chloropus*	More CC when females related	Gibbons, 1986
Temminck's stint *Calidris temminckii*	NKD	Hilden, 1975
Black-headed gull *Larus ridibundus*	More CC in captivity	van Rhijn & Groothuis, 1985
Ring-billed gull *Larus delawarensis*	CC when sex ratio female biased; NKD	LaGrenade & Mousseau, 1983; Conover *et al.*, 1979; Kovacs & Ryder, 1983
Kestrel *Faclo tinnunculus tinnunculus*	NKD	Jourdain, 1926a
Sparrow hawk *Accipiter nisus nisus*	NKD	Jourdain, 1926a; Greeves, 1926
Orange footed scrub fowl *Megapodius reinwardt*	CC when food and incubation foliage sparse	Crome & Brown, 1979
Acorn woodpecker *Melanerpes formicivorus*	More CC when acorns & storage more available; more CC when territories limited	Koenig *et al.*, 1984; Stacey & Koenig, 1984; Mumme *et al.*, 1988
Groove-billed ani *Crotophaga sulcirostris*	CC when more vegetative cover; more CC when habitat saturated	Vehrencamp, 1978; Koford *et al.*, 1986
Speckled mousebird *Colius strictus*	NKD	Decoux, 1982
Splendid fairy wren *Malurus splendens*	NKD	Payne *et al.*, 1988
Eastern chipping sparrow *Spizella passerina passerina*	NKD	Walkinshaw, 1959

Table 3.8. (*cont.*)

Species	Differences in circumstances (CC – when communal care, PC – when parental care, NKD signifies no known difference in circumstances	References
House finch *Carpodacus mexicanus frontalis*	NKD	Michener, 1925
European starling *Sturnus vulgaris*	CC when few nest sites available	Stouffer *et al.*, 1988
Deer mouse *Peromyscus maniculatus*	NKD	Eisenberg, 1968
Vole *Microtus arvalis*	CC when population density increases	Frank, 1957
Brown hyena *Hyaena brunnea*	CC when in clan; PC when solitary	Owens & Owens, 1978, 1979a; Mills, 1982
Red fox *Vulpes vulpes*	CC when co-resident females in a territory lack clear dominance organization	MacDonald, 1979, 1980
Domestic cat *Felis domesticus*	NKD	MacDonald *et al.*, 1987

remain in their parents' territory and care for younger siblings because they have no place to go. This is the habitat saturation hypothesis. A habitat is said to be saturated if all the environment that would support reproduction by members of a particular species is so completely occupied by members of that species that dispersing young adults would be unable to breed. Selander (1964) suggested that habitat saturation was a precondition to helpers at the nest. Brown (1978) and Stacey (1979a) followed this lead in analyzing instances of helpers at the nest. Brown (1987) presented a model of habitat saturation.

These explanations are not mutually exclusive. Each may apply in particular situations, and both may apply in still other cases. The costs and benefits involved are often hard to quantify; consequently, particular instances of helping are interpreted differently by different authors. For example, Wilson (1975) presented helping in Florida scrub jays (*Aphelocoma coerulescens*) as a premier exemplar of kinship selected behavior. But Woolfenden and his associates, who have reported most of the data,

Table 3.9.   *Helpers at the nest and no helpers as alternative parental systems.*

Species	Differences in circumstances (H – when helpers occur, N – when helpers absent, NKD signifies no known difference in circumstances)	References
Cichlid *Lamprologus brichardi*	NKD	Taborsky & Limberger, 1981
Australian little grebe (Dabchick) *Tachybaetus novaehollandiae*	NKD	Lane, 1978
Black swan *Cygnus atratus*	NKD	Braithwaite, 1981
Eider *Somateria mollissima*	H when gull predation high	Ahlen & Andersson, 1970
Purple gallinule *Gallinula martinica*	NKD	Krekorian, 1978
Purple gallinule *Porphyrula martinica*	H when habitat saturated; NKD	Hunter, 1987a,b
Pukeko *Porphyrio porphyrio*	More H in larger territories	Craig, 1984
Osprey *Pandion haliaetus*	H where population density high?	Ogden, 1977
Harris' hawk *Parabuteo unicinctus*	NKD, H not conclusively demonstrated H where large, elusive prey available	Bednarz, 1987; Bednarz & Ligon, 1988
Richardson's merlin *Falco columbarius*	H when population density high (but habitat not saturated)	James & Oliphant, 1986
Black-headed gull *Larus ridibundus*	NKD	van Rhijn & Groothuis, 1985
Southern lapwing *Vanellus chilensis*	NKD	Walters, 1982
Acorn woodpecker *Melanerpes formicivorus*	H when 1) habitat saturated, 2) food production high, 3) stable food facilitates year-round home range; H less common in newly founded groups; More H when acorn crop more reliable; NKD, but acorns or storage not related to H; H where high quality territories not available; more H when group members closer kin?	MacRoberts & MacRoberts, 1976; Stacey, 1979a,b; Stacey & Bock, 1978; Koenig *et al.*, 1984; Stacey & Koenig, 1984; Trail, 1980; Kattan, 1988; Stacey & Ligon, 1987

Table 3.9. (*cont.*)

Species	Differences in circumstances (H – when helpers occur, N – when helpers absent, NKD signifies no known difference in circumstances)	References
Red-cockaded woodpecker *Picoides borealis*	More H with more food	Lennartz *et al.*, 1987
Kookaburra *Dacelo novaeguineae*	Possibly H when population density high	Parry, 1973
Mourning dove *Zenaida macroura*	NKD	Blockstein, 1986
Pied kingfisher *Ceryle rudis rudis*	H when foraging flights longer and fish smaller	Reyer, 1980
Red-throated bee-eater *Merops bullocki*	NKD	Fry, 1972; Crick & Fry, 1986
Grey-crowned babbler *Pomatostomus temporalis*	NKD	Brown *et al.*, 1978
Crested shriketit *Falcunculus frontalus*	NKD	Howe & Noske, 1979
Northwestern crow *Corvus kaurinus*	H in food rich territories	Zerbek & Butler, 1981
Fish crow *Corvus ossifragus*	NKD	McNair, 1985
American crow *Corvus brachyrhynchos*	NKD	Kilham, 1984
Azure-winged magpie *Cyanopica cyana*	NKD	Komeda *et al.*, 1987
Beechey jay *Cyanocorax beecheii*	Possibly H when habitat saturated	Raitt *et al.*, 1984
Common grackle *Quiscalus quiscala*	NKD	Howe, 1979
Speckled mousebird *Colius strictus*	NKD	Decoux, 1982, 1983
Tufted titmouse *Parus bicolor*	NKD	Tarbell, 1983
Pygmy nuthatch *Sitta pygmea*	NKD	Norris, 1958
Brown treecreeper *Climacteris picumnus*	NKD	Noske, 1980
Rufous treecreeper *Climacteris rufa*	NKD	Noske, 1980

Table 3.9.   (*cont.*)

Species	Differences in circumstances (H – when helpers occur, N – when helpers absent, NKD signifies no known difference in circumstances)	References
Red-browed treecreeper *Climacteris erythrops*	NKD	Noske, 1980
Black-tailed treecreeper *Climacteris melanura*	NKD	Noske, 1980
Stripe-backed wren *Campylorhynchus nuchalis*	Possibly more H when fewer breeding opportunities	Rabenold, 1984
Splendid fairy wren *Malurus splendens*	NKD	Payne *et al.*, 1984, 1988
Bicolored wren *Campylorhynchus griseus*	H where population density high	Austad & Rabenold, 1985
Black-capped donacobius *Donacobius atricapillus*	H when habitat saturated	Kiltie & Fitzpatrick, 1984
Rufous hornero *Furnorius rufus*	NKD	Fraga, 1979
Firewood-gatherer *Anumbius*	NKD	Fraga, 1979
Grey-backed fiscal shrike *Lanius excubitorius*	H where habitat saturated	Zack, 1986
Chalk-browed mockingbird *Mimus saturincus*	NKD	Fraga, 1979
Galapagos mockingbird *Nesomimus parvulus*	H more likely if kin present	Curry, 1988
Anteating chat *Myrmecocichla formicivora*	NKD	Earle & Herholdt, 1986
White-browed sparrow *Plocepasser mahali*	NKD	Lewis, 1982
Pied starling *Spreo bicolor*	NKD	Craig, 1987
Bay-winged cowbird *Molothrus badius*	NKD	Fraga, 1972
Bobolink *Dolichonyx oryzivorus*	NKD	Beason & Trout, 1984; Bollinger *et al.*, 1986

Table 3.9.   (*cont.*)

Species	Differences in circumstances (H – when helpers occur, N – when helpers absent, NKD signifies no known difference in circumstances)	References
Brown hyena *Hyaena brunnea*	H in lower productivity habitat; females provisioned all, males provisioned kin	Skinner, 1976; Owens & Owens, 1979a,b; 1984a; Mills, 1982
Black-backed jackal *Canis mesomelas*	NKD	Moehlman, 1979; Ferguson *et al.*, 1983
Red fox *Vulpes vulpes*	H when sex ratio female biased?; H when more food in male territory; NKD	MacDonald, 1979, 1981; Kolb, 1986
Prairie vole *Microtus ochrogaster*	More H at low population density	Getz *et al.*, 1987

held firmly to the habitat saturation hypothesis (e.g., Woolfenden & Fitzpatrick, 1984).

3.7   DETERMINANTS

The best parental-care strategy depends strongly on what others are doing. If a given set of offspring needs a given set of resources for optimum growth and survival, the percentage of those resources any one individual ought to provide will depend on the percentage others are providing. Each care-giver should be trying to provide only enough to fill in the remaining needs of the young. Therefore, a game theoretic approach is particularly valuable in analyzing the determinants of these alternative care-giving systems. Houston & Davies (1985) found that a model developed by the game theoretic approach fitted well the division of parental effort in polyandrous trios of dunnocks.

Ecological circumstances also appear to be powerful determinants. Increased food abundance is sometimes associated with the appearance of helpers at the nest in otherwise parental species, such as the north-western crow (*Corvus kaurinus*). Northwestern crows express two-parent care in inland territories but frequently have helpers at the nest in food-rich coastal territories (Zerbek & Butler, 1981). The fitness contribution of helpers at the nest has been intensively studied (e.g., see Brown, 1987

Table 3.10.   *Two-parent care and one-parent care as alternative parental systems.*

Species	Differences in circumstances (PC – when paternal care given, NP – when no paternal care given, NM – when no maternal care given, NKD signifies no known difference in circumstances)	References
Cichlid *Cichlasoma panamense*	More PC when fewer predators, more females	Townshend & Wootton, 1985
Black swan *Cygnus atratus*	NKD	Braithwaite, 1981
Killdeer *Charadrius vociferus*	NM second clutch	Bunni, 1959; Lenington, 1980
Snowy plover *Charadrius alexandrinus*	PC when nest success & population density high	Warriner *et al.*, 1986
Dotterel *Charadrius morinellus*	NKD	Kalas, 1986
Sanderling *Calidris alba*	NKD	Parmelee & Payne, 1973; Pienkowski & Green, 1976
Snail kite *Rostrhamus sociabilis*	More NP when more food	Beissinger, 1986
California quail *Callipepla californica*	NM when increased plant productivity	McMillan, 1964; Francis, 1965; Leopold, 1977
Ruffed grouse *Bonasa umbellus*	NKD	Hoff, 1984
Blue jay *Cyanocitta cristata*	NKD	Laine, 1981
Long-billed marsh wren *Telmatodyte palustris paludicola* & *T. p. plescies*	More food, less PC	Verner, 1964
Marsh warbler *Acrocephalus palustris*	NKD	Dowsett-Lemaire, 1979
Indigo bunting *Passerina cyanea*	More PC when males older, clutches larger; less PC when polygynous	Westneat, 1988a,b
Bobolink *Dolichonyx oryzivorus*	PC when secondary brood large	Martin, 1974

Table 3.10.   (*cont.*)

Species	Differences in circumstances (PC – when paternal care given, NP – when no paternal care given, NM – when no maternal care given, NKD signifies no known difference in circumstances)	References
Red-winged blackbird *Agelaius phoeniceus*	NKD	Muldal *et al.*, 1986
Brown hyena *Hyaena brunnea*	No PC when more food & communal suckling	Mills, 1982; Owens & Owens, 1979a
Deer mouse *Peromyscus maniculatus*	PC when high overwintering populations	Mihok, 1979
Meadow vole *Microtus pennsylvanicus*	Less PC when housed near other male in lab	Storey & Snow, 1987

for an extended review). While helpers are by no means always helpful, there are circumstances in which they increase the reproductive success of parents. Helpers are often close relatives which benefit via inclusive fitness, and, for example, an improved chance of inheriting a territory.

3.8   HABITAT SATURATION

Habitat saturation is perhaps the most widely cited ecological determinant of helpers at the nest (e.g., Woolfenden & Fitzpatrick, 1984). Stacey (1979b) argued that habitat saturation was the determinant of communal breeding in acorn woodpeckers in the Arizona population he studied. However, Stacey & Ligon (1987) interpreted the results of a long-term investigation as not supporting the habitat saturation hypothesis. Their study revealed that low quality territories were often empty while breeding age birds served as helpers in their parent's territory. The only potential payoff for the helpers was through inclusive fitness.

Whether or not habitat saturation was a factor in this situation depends on how it is defined. If it is defined as there being no place at all to nest, then Stacy & Ligon's work demonstrates that helping occurs in the absence of habitat saturation. However, the birds that bred in the low quality territories without first helping in their parents territory had low

Table 3.11. *Brood reared together as alternative to splitting brood between parents.*

Species	Differences in circumstances (BT – brood reared together, BS – brood split, NKD signifies no known difference in circumstances)	References
Great crested grebe *Podiceps cristatus*	BS when brood size is two or more chicks, earlier if food scarce	Simmons, 1974
Red-necked grebe *Podiceps grisegena* (*grisegena*)	BS when breed on large populated lakes with homogeneous emergent vegetation belts	Wobus, 1964; Chamberlin, 1977
Killdeer *Charadrius vociferus*	NKD	Lenington, 1980
Sandwich tern *Sterna sandvicensis*	NKD	Smith, 1975
Medium ground finch *Geospiza fortis*	More BS when food scarce	Price & Gibbs, 1987
Cactus finch *Geospiza scandens*	More BS when food scarce	Price & Gibbs, 1987
Robin *Erithacus rubecula*	BS when food scarce	Harper, 1985

lifetime direct fitness. Birds that first helped in the parents' territory and later bred in poorer territories, thus adding to their fitness through inclusive fitness, had higher total fitness. Therefore, Stacy & Ligon demonstrated that helping occurred when there was no place better to go than remaining in the parents' territory. If, however, habitat saturation is defined as a situation where only low quality territories are available, then saturation has a role as a determinant of helping. Saturation can be defined either way, but, as the Stacey & Ligon study made clear, the choice of definition is crucial in interpreting the data.

The care-giving system of brown hyenas (*Hyaena brunnea*) similarly varies. In the southern Kalahari desert it is parental in the lower quality but occasionally communal in the higher quality territories (Mills, 1982). It is, however, consistently communal in the central Kalahari (Owens & Owens, 1979a). The ecological determination of this difference may be complex. The increased prey in the central Kalahari may have produced an increased predator population, which raised the likelihood of predation on brown hyena cubs. Consequently, collecting the cubs at a single location may have had an antipredator advantage. Communal care might have developed secondarily. Helpers at the den in silver-backed (*Canis mesomelas*) and golden jackals (*Canis aureus*) appear to make their contributions to the survival of their younger siblings primarily by defending the young from predators while the parents are hunting, although they also feed them (Moehlman, 1986).

Predator pressure appears to be the determinant of communal care in the groove-billed ani (*Crotophaga sulcirostris*) as, when predator pressure is low the monogamous pairs nest separately and maintain territories. The absence of known kinship relations in communal groups strongly suggests predator pressure is the sole determinant of communal breeding (Vehrencamp, 1978).

On the other hand, helping or communal behavior has sometimes appeared when foraging conditions were worse than they were for populations that manifested a parental system. Juvenile helpers occurred in one of two colonies of pied kingfishers (*Ceryle rudis*) (Reyer, 1980). Parents in the colony that had to make longer flights with smaller fish to feed their young, and so were more stressed, had helpers, while parents in the other colony had no helpers (Reyer, 1984). Communal care appeared in the mound building orange footed scrub fowl (*Megapodius reinwardt*) in an area with little vegetation to build into a mound where eggs were incubated by fermentation. Some pairs shared their mound, and hence the exceptionally heavy work of gathering vegetation under those conditions, with a neighboring pair of birds (Crome & Brown, 1979) (see chapter 6). Given the amount of time and energy mound building and maintenance required, the benefits of reduced work load and enhanced reproductive prospects might more than balance such costs as disrupted laying and broken eggs.

3.9   ONE-PARENT AND TWO-PARENT SYSTEMS: background

Trivers (1972) provided a rigorous analysis of the genetic interests of the parents. His analysis made it clear that in many situations each parent could maximize its benefit-cost ratio by minimizing its own care-giving. This adjustment of its care-giving relative to its partner's can take many forms. The most extreme form is to completely cease parental care, leaving the partner to care for the young. This perspective predicts that each parent may try to abandon the young as soon as they can be cared for by only one parent. Such a pre-emptive abandonment strategy has been observed in some species (e.g., Florida snail kites, *Rostrhamus sociabilis* (Beissinger, 1986)).

3.10   ECOLOGICAL DETERMINANTS OF VARIATION IN ONE- AND TWO-PARENT SYSTEMS

An increase in available food is one circumstance in which a one-parent system appears as an alternative to two-parent systems. Male long-billed marsh wrens (*Telmatodytes palustris*) of a subspecies living in a more food-rich environment give less care than males of a different subspecies living where there are scarcer food resources. (Verner, 1964). This one-parent alternative may increase male success by increasing the likelihood of polygynous matings. (In general, circumstances that favor monogamy will favor two-parent systems.) When winter snows confine the activity of mice and increase their loss of body heat (Howard, 1950), the two-parent care may replace the one-parent care system. Under these circumstances males sometimes cohabit with a mate and the young that have been produced, caring for the young (Mihok, 1979). This shift may be a by-product of greater winter gregariousness as a means to minimize heat loss in cold weather.

In some cases polygyny produces both a one-parent and a two-parent system when the male is parental to the young of the primary female but not to the young of secondary females. An example of this is seen in polyterritorial pied flycatchers.

One-parent care replaces two-parent care when female killdeer (*Charadrius vociferus*) abandon their second clutch of young (Lenington, 1980). Lenington supposed these females were in poor physical condition because of the high reproductive investment, and the alternative parental care system was a female adaptation to enhance longevity. Differences in food abundance appear to determine the expression of brood split in at least some cases. Brood-splitting has been reported in the great crested grebe (*Podiceps cristatus*) (Simmons, 1974) and the red-necked grebe (*P. grisegena*) (Wobus, 1964). It occurred when food was less dense or less patchy than was the case when two-parent care was observed. Two-parent care has the advantage of pooling the parental contribution to the young. This assures the more viable young are supported fully by both parents. There would be compensating advantages to splitting the brood when the distribution of food was such that two-parent care involved great inefficiencies in food gathering or transport. Brood split is determined by food abundance somewhat differently in ground finches. When food is abundant males do most of the feeding, and the female may renest or lay a new clutch of eggs while the male rears the current fledglings. But when food is scarce, the brood is divided and each parent rears part of it (Price & Gibbs, 1987).

The intensity and nature of predation might act as a determinant of alternative care systems. For example, under at least some circumstances a two-parent system would be favoured over a one-parent system if the rate of predation on young is high. In a two-parent system one parent could guard all the young, and benefit from an economy of scale.

4

Environmental determinants of intraspecific variation in social systems

Social systems appear to be determined by at least three classes of correlates: ecological, demographic and the social strategies of interacting conspecifics. These three classes of variables seem likely to determine the social system expressed. Moreover, each seems likely to be a broad influence and to be reasonably equally cited as a determinant in empirical analyses of social system variation. To date, that has not happened. Few reports of intraspecific variation in social systems point to the strategy pursued by conspecifics as a determinant of the observed social system. It appears that, rightly or wrongly, most investigators have seen ecological or demographic factors as the priority determinants. The work of Davies (1978, 1989) and his colleagues (Davies & Houston, 1983, 1986; Davies & Lundberg, 1984) with dunnocks shows that these determinants can be integrated.

4.1 GAME THEORY

The social strategies being pursued by conspecifics are bound to be major determinants of the success of one's own social strategies. Therefore, the social system expressed will likely be determined in part by the social strategies of others. This compelling logic is the underlying premise of the approach pioneered by Maynard Smith and known as the game theory approach. The fact that the success of an individual's strategy depends on the strategies others might employ tends to select for a social strategy that will confer high fitness whatever strategy others might employ. Since such strategies are favored by selection they should be stable in evolutionary time. They have come to be called Evolutionarily Stable Strategies (Maynard Smith, 1976, 1982).

This perspective has been successfully employed by Davies & Houston (1986) in their analysis of parental care in dunnocks. Breeding dunnocks are organized both as monogamous pairs and as trios composed of one female and two males. This difference in social systems is attributed to an ecological variable – the distribution and abundance of food (see chapter 3). When a female confines her home range to the territory of a particular male, the pair breeds monogamously. But the female may establish a home range that includes the territories of two males. These two territories will gradually merge into one defended by both males, who will form a dominant–subordinate dyad. In some of the trios thus formed both males will copulate with the female and so form a polyandrous mating group.

For the dunnock, a parental-care system develops from the mating system. The female lays and incubates a set of eggs. (If she is copulating with two males she lays more eggs than if she is copulating with only one.) When the chicks are hatched the mother begins to feed them; in polyandrous trios both males also feed the young, while in nonpolyandrous trios only the male who has copulated feeds the young.

The game theory approach suggests that the investment a male parent makes should be determined, in part, by what the other individual is doing. In fact, the feeding behavior of a breeding male is determined by both the number of young to be fed and whether or not a second male is feeding. Thus the behavior of one animal has been in part determined by the behavioral strategy of another.

4.2   ECOLOGICAL DETERMINANTS

In the literature to date, game theory has not had a prominent role. Most instances of intraspecific variation in social systems have been analyzed as determined directly by ecological variables, along the lines of interspecific socioecology. One component of socioecology has involved studies and hypotheses matching an array of ecological circumstances with an array of social systems. Through this matching process a number of ecological circumstances that may have determined social systems over evolutionary time have been identified. Table 4.1 relates a number of proposed determinants to the social systems they have been shown (or proposed) to determine.

The analysis of the ecological determinants of social system variation has drawn upon those matches and has assigned a number of those determinants the same role in intraspecific variation. For the most part the determinants seem to work well in their new role. However, the determination of social systems over evolutionary time differs from their determination over ecological space or time in ways that make wholesale transfer of these variables inappropriate.

Table 4.1A.   *Predicted ecological correlates of intraspecific variation in social systems.*

Predicted correlates	
Ecological correlate	Reference
Food	
Size, abundance, spatial and temporal distribution	
Group vs. solitary living	
Homogeneous prey distribution → pairs	MacDonald, 1983
Increase prey size (carnivores) → increase group size	
Rich habitat → increase group size	
Cyclic prey availability → change group size	
Large prey, open habitat, high population density → group	Packer, 1986
Increase food abundance → let offspring stay → increase group size	von Schantz, 1984
Decrease food → evict offspring → decrease group size	
Mating systems	
Food abundant → mate desertion → serial polygamy	Beissinger, 1986
Distribution, density	
Group vs. solitary living	
Increase food density → decrease searching → increase aggression → group to solitary	Caraco, 1979a
Spacing systems	
Superabundant food → no territory	Myers *et al.*, 1981
Very low food density → no territory	
Intermediate food density → no territory	
Cooperative breeding	
High reliable acorn production → cooperative breeding	Trail, 1980
Low, unreliable acorn production → no cooperative breeding	
High oak diversity → high crop reliability → larger woodpecker units, more storage holes	
Predation	
Group vs. solitary living	
Concentrated predators → group	Rubenstein, 1986
Habitat/Seasonality	
Mating systems	
Shifts in local food abundance alters mate availability → polyandry or monogamy	Colwell & Oring, 1988

Table 4.1A.   (*cont.*)

Predicted correlates	
Ecological correlate	Reference
Suitable nest sites limited (holes) → polygyny	Roell, 1979
Spatial/temporal variation in breeding habitat → polygyny	Siegfried, 1978
Few suitable nest sites → polygyny	Stouffer *et al.*, 1988
Prairie or mountain, low host nest density, high cowbird density → nonterritorial → promiscuity	Teather & Robertson, 1986
Abundant host nests → females defend territories → males defend females → monogamy or polygyny	
Cooperative breeding	
Few nest sites → cooperative breeding	Gowaty, 1981
Intense nest predation → cooperative breeding	
Lack of suitable nest sites → cooperative breeding	Stouffer *et al.*, 1988
Temperature	
Group vs. solitary living	
Decrease temperature → increase feeding time to maintain homeothermy → decrease aggression → solitary to group	Caraco, 1979a
Resources in general	
Mating systems	
Patchy resources → polygyny	Siegfried, 1978

The social system adjustments analyzed in traditional socioecology are assumed to have taken place over evolutionary time. The history of their adjustment can appropriately be conceptualized as variations in social behavior being selected by natural selection. In this scenario little or no assessment of circumstances by the behavioral phenotype is involved. Variations are simply exposed to natural selection and increase or decrease according to their fitness consequences. Most instances of intraspecific variation in social systems require something that functions like an assessment step. In order to make an adaptive adjustment of social behavior, the behaving individual must assess the ecological circumstances. Not all ecological variables are equally available for assessment. The distribution of food is probably readily assessed by reasonably mobile animals. The density of predator populations and of conspecifics will also usually be salient. On the other hand, the kind and prevalence of

Table 4.1B. *Demonstrated   ecological   correlates   of   intraspecific variation in social systems.*

Demonstrated correlates	
Ecological correlate	Reference
Food	
Size, abundance, spatial and temporal distribution	
Group vs. solitary living	
Small, abundant food source → solitary	Alcock, 1984
Larger prey → group, cooperative hunt	
Large prey → group	Bowen, 1981
Small prey → solitary	
Unable to disperse → larger groups	
Larger prey → solitary to group	Caraco & Wolf, 1975
Large, undefendable, unpredictable food clumps → group	Krebs, 1974
Abundant food → group	
Widely scattered and/or easily defendable food → solitary	
Large prey → cooperative hunt → group	Kruuk, 1975
Widely scattered, small food → solitary	
Increased prey biomass → increased group size	Kruuk & Parish, 1987
Increased patch quality (amount of food/ patch) → increased group size	
Low food availability → solitary	
Abundant, patchy food → group size	MacDonald, 1981
Uniformly dispersed prey → decrease group size	
Small prey, sparsely distributed → solitary	Owens & Owens, 1978
Large carcass → concentrated food → group	
Highly clumped food at any given time → group	Smith, 1977
Distribution, density	
Large clumped prey → increase food available → increase group size	Bekoff & Wells, 1980
Abundant food, clumped, defendable → solitary to group	Bekoff *et al.*, 1984
Richness food patch → group size	
Increase prey biomass → solitary to group	Caraco & Wolf, 1975
Low starvation risk → solitary to group	Ekman & Hake, 1988
Small, dispersed resources, ripe for long time → small group or solitary	Klein & Klein, 1977
Fast ripening fruit, scattered → large group	
Patchy, unpredictable food → colonial nest	Krebs, 1974
Large patches food, water → decrease competition → group	Rubenstein, 1986
Food type	
Carrion → large, clumped food source → group	Bekoff & Wells, 1980
Rodents → not defendable food → solitary	

Table 4.1B. (*cont.*)

Demonstrated correlates	
Ecological correlate	Reference
Larger prey patches → solitary to group	Malcolm, 1986
Spacing systems	
Concentrated prey → small female home range → males defend area	Caro & Collins, 1986
Low numbers of prey → large female home ranges → males do not defend area	
Low flower abundance → not territorial	Carpenter & MacMillen, 1976
High flower abundance → not territorial	
Intermediate flower abundance → territorial	
Seasonally high resource production, good breeding habitat → permanent territory	Craig, 1979
Year-round food separated from high production of food → seasonal territory	
Superior winter food near territory → partial breakdown of territoriality	
Heterogeneity between and within habitats → not territorial	
Abundant food → increase intruder pressure → abandon territory	Davies, 1976
Scarce food → abandon territory	
Dispersed food in small area → tight flock	
Food spread in large area → loose flock	
Food concentrated in small clumps → territorial	
Predictable food, prey renewal → permanent territory	
No dry winter forage, food available elsewhere → not territorial, migratory	Franklin, 1983
Scattered clumps of preferred, productive food → feeding territory	
Intermediate nectar levels → territorial	Gill & Wolf, 1975
High nectar levels → not territorial	
Widely scattered food and/or easily defendable → territorial	Krebs, 1974
Increased food availability → territorial	Kruuk & Parish, 1987
Stable, predictable food → large feeding/nesting territory	Walsberg, 1977
Ephemeral food → colonial	
Mating systems	
Increased prey abundance → polygyny	Hamerstrom *et al.*, 1985
Decreased prey abundance → monogamy	
Large homogeneous territories → monogamy	Osborne & Bourne, 1977

Table 4.1B.   (*cont.*)

Demonstrated correlates	
Ecological correlate	Reference
Small heterogeneous territories → simultaneous polyandry	
Cooperative breeding	
Capture large, elusive prey → immatures do not disperse, birds live in groups, cooperate in prey capture → cooperative breeding	Bednarz & Ligon, 1988
Mates	
Spacing systems	
Receptive females unpredictable resource → not territorial	Erlinge & Sandell, 1986
Predation	
Group vs. solitary living	
Scavenger pressure → solitary to group	Caraco & Wolf, 1975
Lower predation risk → solitary	Elgar, 1986
Mating systems	
High nest predation → concentrate in protected areas → dense population → increase polyandry	Oring & Lank, 1986
Heavy predation → monogamy	Osborne & Bourne, 1977
Light predation → simultaneous polyandry	
High predation rate → polyandry	Petrie, 1986
Parental care systems	
High predation → more paternal	Petrie, 1986
Temperature	
Group vs. solitary living	
Low temperature → increase feeding requirement → decrease aggression → solitary to group	Caraco, 1979b
Increase temperature → increase aggression → group to solitary	
Decrease temperature → increase time feeding → solitary to group	Elgar, 1986
Low temperature → flock	Emlen, 1952
Climate	
Spacing systems	
Food limiting at end of dry season → year-round territory	Richard, 1974
Habitat	
Group vs. solitary living	
Increase frequency of favored habitat patches → increase group size	Brown & Balda, 1977

Table 4.1B.   (*cont.*)

Demonstrated correlates	
Ecological correlate	Reference
Increase home range cover → increase group size	
Increase amount of herbaceous cover, tree cover → increase group size	
Dispersion of cover → group size	Brown *et al.*, 1983
Hard soil → hard to dig warrens → large, cohesive groups	Cowan & Garson, 1985
Light soil → simple warrens → no tight groups	
Complex suburban habitat → hard to set up clear boundaries → solitary to group	Kolb, 1986
Uniform habitat → pairs	MacDonald, 1983
Rich, diverse habitat → increase group size	
Nest sites	
High competition for nest sites → communal breeding	Craig, 1979
Few nest sites → colonial	Simmons, 1970
Spacing systems	
Low plankton level → territorial	Fricke, 1977
Higher plankton level → not territorial	
Variable cover for nest sites → defend sites	Petrie, 1986
Prairie habitat → low host nest density, high cowbird density → not territorial	Teather & Robertson, 1986
Abundant host nests → territorial	
Human dwellings → stable food → territory	Zahavi, 1971
Mating systems	
Harsh, unproductive areas → sparsely distributed resources → indefensible → monogamy	Flinn & Low, 1986
Limited home sites → polygyny	Fricke, 1977
Breed in simple habitats → breeding pairs dispersed → serial monogamy	Osborne & Bourne, 1977
Limited nest sites and food abundance → polygyny	Quinney, 1983
Homogeneous area → burrows not clustered → tend to monogamy	Roberts, 1987
Cooperative breeding	
Stable environment → cooperative breeding	Craig, 1979
Differences in territory quality → cooperative breeding	
Heterogeneity within and between habitats → cooperative breeding	
Habitat saturated → cooperative breeding	Woolfenden & Fitzpatrick, 1986

Table 4.1B.   (*cont.*)

Demonstrated correlates	
Ecological correlate	Reference
Resources in general	
Spacing systems	
Unpredictable, variable resource distribution → no defense	Myers *et al.*, 1981
Evenly dispersed, stable resources → territorial	
Mating systems	
Immobile or limited resource → control distribution → polyandry	Flinn & Low, 1986
Surplus resources → males control → unequal distribution → polygyny	

diseases and parasites may be important determinants of social systems (Alexander, 1974; Freeland, 1976) and may vary greatly over ecological time, but in many cases it may be difficult to perceive them and to assess their impact.

The fact that intraspecific variation is produced by mechanisms is an additional difference between it and traditional socioecology. Some cases of intraspecific variation will be maladaptive because the mechanisms will work imperfectly. The assessment procedure has some probability of failure, and the mechanisms that produce change may also fail. This expectation of intraspecific socioecology differs from the assumptions of interspecific socioecology. Of course, interspecific socioecology encountered examples of social systems that seemed maladaptive. In fact these maladaptations led to explanations involving phylogenetic inertia. Even so, phylogenetic inertia would never be called on to explain a shift from an adaptive pattern to a maladaptive one in unchanging circumstances, although such a social system shift could take place intraspecifically through accumulation of mechanical errors.

4.3   ECOLOGICAL VARIABLES

4.3.1   Predation

Variation in the kind and intensity of predation can act as a determinant of several kinds of social systems. A change in the intensity of predator pressure may determine a change between solitary and group living. Group living imposes many costs. One of its clearest benefits, however, is increased efficiency in the management of predation pressure (Hamilton, 1971; Bertram, 1978). The members of wood pigeon (*Columba palumbus*) flocks feed more efficiently when in groups than when solitary because of reduced time spent on predator alert (Kenward, 1978). Fish in schools are less vulnerable to predation than solitary fish (Neill & Cullen, 1974).

The form predator pressure takes should also influence the value of social groups. Black-headed gulls in colonies on an exposed beach had more reproductive success than gulls nesting solitarily when subject to carrion crow predation (Patterson, 1965). In contrast, brown-hooded gulls in a colony had lower reproductive success than brown-hooded gulls nesting solitarily when subject to caracara predation (Burger, 1974). This difference appears to be due to the differences in predator behavior. Carrion crows hunt alone, while caracaras hunt in pairs. Mobbing birds rising from their nests to attack the solitary carrion crow effectively shelter their nests from predation, but mobbing birds rising from their nests to attack the first of a pair of caracaras entering the colony leave their nests exposed to the second member of the pair which enters below the mobbing birds. Under such predation pressure crypsis, facilitated by the availability of high marsh grass, is a better strategy, and solitary pairs are more cryptic.

Variations in predator pressure can also act as a determinant of variations in parental care systems. Helpers at the nest reduced the rate of predation on silver-backed jackal pups (Moehlman, 1986). Whether or not helpers pay their costs could vary as a function of predator intensity. Communal nesting in groove billed ani appears to be driven in good part by the level of nest predation, since pairs exposed to less predator pressure are less likely to nest communally (Vehrencamp, 1978).

4.3.2   Food Distribution

Another major ecological determinant of social systems is the distribution of food. Brown (1964) pointed out that a key to understanding territoriality is the concept of economic defensibility of resources. Food as a resource is most economically defended when its distribution is patchy. Therefore, the existence of foraging territories ought to be, and is, determined in great part by the patchiness of food. As a consequence intraspecific variation between territoriality and an undefended home range is often attributable to the patchiness with which food is distributed in a territory. Burros (*Eguus asinus*) live in a range of habitats where a substantial food reserve is concentrated at a particular site, e.g., along a stretch of riparian habitat, a male may defend the patch as a territory. Where food is less concentrated, e.g., in a desert, all individuals live in undefended home ranges (Woodward, 1979).

The patchiness of food distribution can act as a determinant of breeding systems as well. The fact that concentrated resources permit one individual to economically defend enough food for several individuals means that individual can hold the resources for several mates. Thus, males may be able to express polygyny rather than monogamy, and females may be able to express polyandry rather than monogamy in areas where the resources are more patchily distributed.

Animals breeding in exceptionally rich food patches may also manifest different parental care systems. When one parent is able to control a rich source of food, the other parent may be able to care for the young without help. If one parent ceases to help, a one-parent system is expressed. Often a change from a two-parent to a one-parent system accompanies a change from a monogamous to a polygamous system. An example of such a double shift was observed in long-billed marsh wrens (*Cistothorus elatensis*) breeding in a poor versus rich food habitat (Verner, 1964).

4.3.3   Stability of food distribution

The stability of the distribution of food in space can affect social systems related to food. Phainopepla (*Phainopepla nitens*) defends an all-purpose territory when it breeds in the desert and forages on mistletoe berries. On the other hand, when it feeds on buckthorn, in more moist habitats, it defends only a small space around its nest (Walsberg, 1977). The crucial difference appears to be that the mistletoe have a long fruiting season, so the berries represent a reliable and inexhaustible food source throughout the breeding season. On the other hand, each buckthorn plant fruits for only one or two weeks, then must be abandoned for another. An even more ephemeral food source is a large school of fish in the ocean. Parasitic jaegers nest in colonies when they feed by stealing fish from other seabirds that harvest schooling fish, while the same species feeding on lemmings nest in all-purpose territories (Pitelka *et al.*, 1955; Andersson & Gotmark, 1980). (It is not clear what the advantages of the colony are. Perhaps the nesting area has favorable air currents.)

4.3.4 Food abundance

The abundance of food can act as a determinant of social systems in several ways. For one thing it can act as a determinant of the economic defensibility of food. As the abundance of food decreases, a point will be reached at which the costs in energy and risk of predation no longer offset the benefits of territory ownership. On the other hand, when the abundance of food becomes high a cost to benefit shift takes place in the same direction because the individual's foraging needs are met so quickly while foraging from undefended sources. The relaxation of territoriality in the face of superabundance of food has been observed in the golden-winged and bronzy sunbirds (*Nectarinia killimensis*) (Gill & Wolf, 1975; Wolf, 1978; Lott & Lott, unpubl.) and the iwi (Carpenter & MacMillen, 1976).

The decreased cost of foraging competition with increased food abundance also has the effect of lowering the cost of group living, which has several potential consequences for social systems. Decreased food competition may facilitate a shift from solitary to group living. The lower cost of group living may also affect breeding systems and parental care systems. For example, if low food competition facilitates group foraging by female mammals it will facilitate defense of a group of females by a single male, and thus facilitate polygyny rather than monogamy (Wrangham, 1986). Similarly, a decreased cost of grouping may facilitate certain forms of communal care of young. California quail sometimes combine very young broods into a super-brood that is tended by all four parents (Mastrup, pers. comm.). This tendency toward communal brood rearing seems to be correlated with high levels of food. California quail are highly precocial. Parental care, even of the newly hatched chicks, consists largely of accompanying the foraging chicks, acting as a guide to food and a sentinel against predators. If food for the chicks is scarce, families are in competition for it. If food is abundant competition is less. Since one parent acts as a sentinel at all times, each of the four parents of a combined brood has only half the sentinel time of each of the two parents of a brood maintained separately.

4.3.5 Physical character of habitat

In some cases the social system expressed appears to be determined by the physical character of the area the species is living in. Ungulates living on open habitat can form and maintain groups more easily than those in forests (Barrette, 1988). The configuration of the area may also be important. The costs of territorial defense are lowered when some of the boundaries do not need to be defended. While feral horses (*Equus caballus*) are not normally territorial, part of the population living on an island are territorial (Rubenstein, 1986). In this situation the land mass is long and narrow, and the territories have short boundaries across the length of the area. Consequently, most of the territorial boundary is shoreline which can be defended inexpensively. Such a reduction in the cost of territorial defense may have other ramifications. Dippers limit their activity to riparian habitat. During the breeding season the animals are territorial. A population studied by Price & Bock (1973) had a set of linear territories along a stream in Colorado. Each male's resource defense probably emphasized the boundaries between territories. The males at the ends of the series of territories had to defend only one boundary. Those males had larger territories, and each of them bred polygynously, while all the males with two territorial neighbors bred monogamously.

4.3.6   Climate

Climatic variables may determine intraspecific variation in social systems in several ways. A factor particularly important for temperate zone species is the length of the breeding season. A longer breeding season creates a greater potential for multiple breeding by one sex. Polyandry in red phalaropes (Schamel & Tracy, 1977) and polygyny in savannah sparrows (*Passerculus sandwichensis*) (Weatherhead, 1979b) as alternatives to monogamy seem to be due to greater length of breeding season. Extreme climates, such as the polar climates, make seasonal occupancy and migration likely. A migratory population may be more predisposed to female natal philopatry, which in turn may predispose them to monogamy with pair formation taking place before migration (McKinney, 1986). A short breeding season will also produce young of similar ages throughout a population. Since these young would have similar needs at any one time, the possibility of communal care might be increased. In the instances of communal care in California quail, the combined broods were always hatched less than a week apart (Mastrup, pers. comm.). On the other hand, where the breeding season is long, there will be less synchrony in the needs of the mothers and infants. This may reduce group size and seems likely to reduce group stability, because females may realign themselves to join groups composed of individuals that have similar physiological needs.

Loss of body heat in cold climates can be a problem and in some species groups function to provide heat for one another. Hyraxes and bob-white quail (*Colinus virgianus*) huddle for warmth during the night. Ligon & Ligon (1988) attributed the communal behavior of the green woodhoopoe (*Phoeniculus purpureus*) in cooler climates to the reduced nocturnal heat loss that occurs when the birds huddle together in hollow trees.

Climate may also affect the social system by its effect on communication. For example, high rainfall may increase the cost of scent marking by rapidly degrading scents. Rapid degradation of scent marks would increase the cost of a territorial system that depended on these scent marks and so tilt the population affected toward a different form of spacing system.

4.3.7 Escape cover-shelter

The kind and abundance of shelter from predation may influence the degree of solitariness in several ways. One effect of cover or shelter is that the more cover or shelter the population has the less the predator pressure is likely to be. Another effect is that many forms of cover are likely to influence group size by influencing the effectiveness of communication and coordination among members of a social group. The usual form of cover for terrestrial vertebrates is provided by the plant community, and correlations between the character of the plant community and the size and nature of social groups have been reported in several species. Female white-tailed deer in a more open habitat are in groups while the same species in closed habitat tend to be solitary (Hirth, 1977). Reedbuck were solitary while living in a dense plant community, but when fire destroyed most of the plant cover, they began to live in groups (Jungius, 1971). Mountain goats (*Oreamus americanus*) are solitary or in very small groups when living on cliffs, but tend to be in larger groups when in flatter habitat, even if both areas are above timberline (Lott, unpubl. obs.). Presumably the steepness of the cliff surroundings offers protection from wolf predation for the rather slow-moving mountain goats.

It is not clear in any of these examples whether the affected individuals are in small groups because they are constrained from getting into larger ones by the high cover, or if they enter larger groups because they have increased predator anxiety when alone in the absence of cover. It is certainly the case that there are costs of belonging to a group, e.g., competition for resources is higher, and competition for resources is increased when the animals are channeled by topography and the physical constraints of the plant community. The narrower the front in which a group can move, the greater the disadvantage for those at the rear of the group in food competition.

4.3.8   Habitat gradient steepness

The steepness of the gradient of the habitat on which a species is dependent may influence the social system expressed. For example, nonmigratory acorn woodpeckers depend on an environment with several features combined. While they are substantially insectivorous during the summer, they depend on stored acorns during the winter. Stored acorns require both oaks to provide the acorns and pine or dead trees to provide the softer bark or wood in which acorn storage holes can be drilled. Consequently their habitat requirements form a steep gradient that constrains dispersal. In these areas the social system they express is communal breeding (MacRoberts & MacRoberts, 1976). On the other hand, when the habitat does not contain the resources needed for overwintering, they mate monogamously and overwinter elsewhere (Stacey & Bock, 1978). Moreover the mating and offspring care systems may vary within a population. Parental care was expressed in territories with low storage capacity, and communal care in territories with high storage facilities (Stacey & Ligon, 1987).

4.3.9   Habitat saturation

The degree to which the habitat is saturated with members of a particular species can act as a determinant of the social system expressed. This variable seems to act primarily by limiting the dispersal of the young. Habitat saturation is the explanation advanced for group living and helpers in the Florida scrub jay (Woolfenden & Fitzpatrick, 1984). In analyses of social ecology of acorn woodpeckers (Koenig *et al.*, 1984), coyotes (Andelt, 1985), and jackals (Moehlman, 1986), this variable has been advanced as an explanation for the retention of young, leading to larger social groups and sometimes to helpers at the nest.

4.3.10   Human persecution

Human persecution of animals may have a number of effects on social systems. In the first place humans may greatly reduce populations by harvesting them. Features of social systems that are a function of high population density may therefore disappear. A population of bobcats

(*Lynx rufus*) subjected to heavy trapping pressure had a relatively low density. This population was organized territorially, while another population not reduced by trapping, and therefore much denser, lived in undefended home ranges (Zezulak & Schwab, 1979). In contrast, the territorial breeding system of a pronghorn antelope population broke down under heavy hunting pressure and the animals bred in dominance organized herds (Copeland, 1980). In coyote populations brought to low density by human persecution, the basic social unit is mated pairs, but solitary individuals, including nomads, are common. In contrast, in an area of high population density (protected from human persecution) parents are much more likely to retain the young (Andelt, 1985).

The removal of large numbers of animals from the population of group living animals will have the immediate effect of reducing the size of groups. Human persecution has influenced breeding in some monk (*Monachus schauinslandi*) and weddell seal (*Leptonychotes weddelli*) populations (Jouventin & Cornet, 1980). In these cases the reduction in group size was so great that the breeding system changed from the characteristic polygyny to monogamy. Some forms of human persecution are experienced as increased predator pressure. If so there will be an opposing force on the animals, encouraging the formation of larger groups. Forming larger groups from smaller groups that have been reduced by hunting, trapping or fishing would decrease the stability of groups.

Human persecution may change the operational sex ratio and thus increase the probability of polygyny. Operational sex ratios may also be altered by general population reduction. For example, female coyotes in a low density population achieve reproductive status in the first rather than their second year. Kleiman (1977) predicted that human persecution will produce polygyny in coyotes.

Most of the effects already discussed are likely to take place over ecological time. There are other effects of human persecution that are more likely to produce their effects over evolutionary time. These effects exploit a feature of the social organization of the persecuted species in such a way that that feature is selected against. Most commercial fisheries concentrate on schooling fish, and fishermen prefer larger schools. This creates a selective pressure against schooling in commercially fished populations, and may reduce the size of schools or even produce solitary behavior in those populations.

Snow geese (*Chen caerulescens*) have strong family loyalties during their first year. If a member of a family is shot by a hunter, the other members of the family are likely to return to the area in search of it, where they are also likely to be shot. This introduces a selective pressure against family loyalty in hunted populations, and may eventually change their social structure (Prevett & MacInnes, 1980).

4.3.11   Pollution

Another form of human impact on social systems is through the introduction of chemicals that alter the behavior of animals directly or indirectly. There are several potential indirect impacts of chemicals. A well-known effect of some pesticides is their concentration at higher trophic levels. In practice this has meant that when a poison is introduced into a community it quickly accumulates most rapidly in the predators.

A disproportionate impact of toxins on the predator component of a community would lower predator pressure, and that would have an impact on the costs and benefits of group living by prey species. Some species are highly responsive to immediate manifestations of predator pressure and their social organization changes in response to these shifts. Wintering sanderlings at Bodega Bay, California defended territories in years when no merlins (*Falco columbarius*) were hunting the beaches, but they were not territorial in winters when a merlin was present (Connors, pers. comm.).

Toxics may also reduce the population density of a species, and that reduction, in turn, may change social systems. The potential for polygamy, communal breeding and helpers at the nest are all greater in higher density populations. A final indirect impact of pollution would be to change the distribution or abundance of food, increasing or decreasing its total biomass or its patchiness. A decrease in total biomass of a food source would decrease the carrying capacity of the environment for the species being considered. The immediate effect of that change would be to increase the degree of habitat saturation, thus inclining some species to a shift toward communal nesting or helpers at the nest or den. The long term effect would be to lower the whole population, thus decreasing the likelihood of social systems related to high populations. A change in the distribution of food resources could have profound effects, as discussed earlier in this chapter.

Toxic chemicals may also have direct effects on behavior. High levels of an insecticide used to control forest pests made juvenile coho salmon (*Onchorhynchus kisutch*) less territorial (Bull & McInerney, 1974). It is not clear how such an impact could occur, but it is likely that some more general behavioral property is disrupted. For example, it is known that some pollutants disrupt the memory of some animals. Certainly the

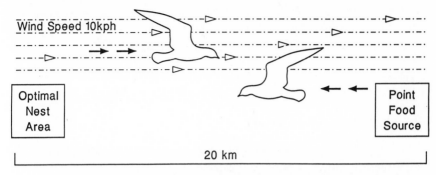

Fig. 4.1. Round trips in a steady wind take more time than the same trips ins till air. The wind is blowing from an optimal nest area to a point source of food at 10 kph, A bird flying 20 kph would have a ground speed of 30 kph (20 kph + 10 kph) outbound with a tailwind and make the trip in 40 min. The return trip ground speed would be 10 kph (20 kph − 10 kph) and take two hours. In contrast each leg of the trip would take one hour in still air for a two hour round trip. In this example, a bird that flew eight hours could make four round trips ins till air, but only three round trips in a 10 kph wind.

ability to memorize landmarks is necessary to territoriality, so a disruption of memory could disrupt territoriality.

4.3.12 Wind

Currents of either air or water increase the costs of social strategies and, therefore, have the potential to alter social systems of animals that fly or swim. The cost is imposed by the fact that a round trip in a steady current of either air or water takes more energy (and usually more time) than the same trip in still air (Lott, in prep.). This is because an outbound trip against a current of either wind or water takes longer and uses more energy than the animal saves on the return trip with the aid of the same current of wind or water, compared to a trip in still air or water. Consequently there is a net cost of making round trips in wind and currents as opposed to still air or water (Fig. 4.1). This net cost changes the energy balance involved in central place foraging and territoriality.

The patterns of global circulation make winds higher in some latitudes (e.g., the roaring forties) than in others (the horse latitudes around 25 degrees north and south of the equator, and at the equator itself). Species whose range includes both windy and calm regions would encounter quite different costs and benefits of central place foraging and territoriality in those different areas. Optimal adjustments to the different cost-benefit ratios created by winds of different strengths would sometimes require the use of dispersed nesting rather than colonial nesting or living in undefended home ranges rather than in territories. The expression of these alternatives under these conditions has not been reported, but a search for them might be profitable.

4.3.13   Disease and parasites

The impact of disease and parasites as ecological or evolutionary pressures shaping either varying or unvarying social systems is little known, but is increasingly discussed. Hart (1988) pointed out that the amount of resources devoted to the operation of the immune system indicates the biological significance of disease and parasites to animals, and he suggested that the use of behavior in support of the immune system in disease and parasite management is likely, e.g., the behavioral response to fever supports an immune system challenged by bacteria. Alexander (1974) pointed out that the risk of getting a disease is likely to impose a limit on sociality in many species. Freeland (1976) reviewed the available literature on the relationship of disease to social behavior in primates and developed the idea of disease and parasites as possible determinants of primate social systems. He has pursued the line of thought in a series of theoretical and empirical papers (Freeland, 1977, 1979, 1980, 1981a,b, 1983). There have been demonstrations that disease acts as a determinant of social status in several dominance organized species (e.g., Rau, 1984), and disease has been shown to produce change in the social organization of Australian magpies (*Gymnorhina tibicen*) (Carrick, 1963). Sticklebacks form larger groups when there are more parasites (Poulin & Fitzgerald, 1989) (Fig. 4.2).

The demonstrated impact of parasites and diseases on social systems is much less than their apparent potential impact. Parasites and diseases are undoubtedly important ecological variables (e.g., May, 1988; Scott, 1988), and it is intuitively compelling to suppose that animals would manage their challenges partly via social behavior. Some aspects of disease management via individual behavior have been rigorously analyzed (Hart, 1988). Hamilton & Zuk (1984) have pointed out that mate selection might well be influenced by disease and parasite loads and resistances. However, neither of these suggestions nor those of Alexander & Freeland have yet been compellingly supported by further findings. One of the reasons must be that the facts of epidemiology often contradict the behaviorist's intuitions about the nature of their ecological impact. Consequently, informed development of this relationship is a few

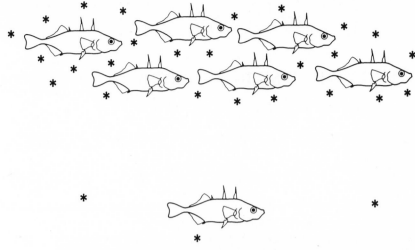

Fig. 4.2. Sticklebacks formed shoals when parasite density was high (Poulin & Fitzgerald, 1989). Shoaling fish may suffer less parasitism per individual via the selfish herd effect. Alternatively, or additionally, they may benefit via increased opportunities to prey on the parasites. Thus the shoal could form partly because its members use one another as reliable indicators of available food.

years in the future. Therefore, I have resisted the temptation to speculate about the role of parasites and diseases in producing intraspecific variation in social systems.

There are many more cases in which variation in an ecological variable has been predicted or shown to act as a determinant of intraspecific variation in one or more social systems (Table 4.1). Predictions of social system variation are usually drawn from the roles of particular variables assigned in socioecological theory. Many have recognized that intraspecific variation in social systems can provide a way to test socioecological hypotheses. This welcome possibility has certain limits, however. Both the potential and its limits are most clearly seen in the context of the proximate mechanisms that must underly particular instances of social system variation (chapters 5 and 6) and social variation as an evolved strategy (chapter 7). Consequently, I have deferred full discussion of this issue to chapter 8.

5

Social system variation
mechanisms: processes

We have seen that the social systems of many vertebrate species vary substantially within the species. Hypotheses about the ecological determinants and adaptiveness of these variations are being readily adapted from the socioecological literature to account for these variations. But a central question has not yet been addressed. What proximate processes produce these adaptive alternatives? It is especially clear in cases of intraspecific variation in social systems that it is not the social systems themselves that have been selected, but the proximate processes that produce them. Discovery of these processes will enrich our understanding of animal behavior and the necessary research will reward generations of scientists.

There are two aspects to the general question of learning about these mechanisms. The first is establishing a conceptual structure. What kinds of processes must operate to produce the social system variation we observe? How do the needs of different social system variation constrain these processes, e.g., how quickly must they operate? What kind of information would the process need to operate adaptively? With these requirements in mind, we can then cast about among known behavioral processes to see which of them might accomplish the ends we have identified within the constraints we have worked out. These conceptual issues are addressed in this chapter.

The second step is to bring this conceptual material to bear on the variations we observe and try to generate hypotheses about how particular sets of social system alternatives could be produced by the processes we have identified in this chapter. Many species alternate between being solitary and being in a group. What processes could account for these alternatives and how do they produce them? Of course, I am unable to answer that question, but I can suggest some possibilities which should at least make the conceptual issues more tangible and may even suggest some research. We need to take the same approach to other sets of alternatives as well. These applications of the conceptual issues raised in this chapter are attempted in the next.

Up to now the mechanisms producing particular instances of intraspecific variation in social systems have seldom been analyzed. Therefore we must draw upon knowledge of phenomena that are already known to change behavior, or that might produce changes in behavior, and see if they make intelligible instances of intraspecific variation in social systems. This section must contain a good bit of speculation, and many of its specific predictions will prove to be wrong. However quickly the predictions fail, they will have served the purpose of making it clear that some mechanism must have operated, and that our understanding of a case of intraspecific variation is not complete until we know what that mechanism is. In doing that alone, they will have served a useful purpose.

5.1   CONCEPTUALIZING SOCIAL SYSTEM VARIATION MECHANISMS

In most cases we will need to think of the mechanisms as consisting of three processes: a process that assesses the individual's ecological or demographic circumstances, a process that chooses which of the available systems to live in and a process of change in pattern of interaction that produces a change from, for example, group to solitary living or vice versa. This conceptual step is an essential precondition to research on an example of this variation, because one research task will be to tease apart the assessment and change the processes in order to test specific hypotheses.

The nature of such mechanisms will be partly revealed by considering what they must do. Social systems are a product of social interactions. Consequently, a change in social systems requires a mechanism that changes social interactions. Therefore, a mechanism must explain changes at the individual level producing alterations in individual behavior.

In addition to accounting for change at the appropriate level, intraspecific variation mechanisms must have properties that make much of the variation in social systems adaptive. For the variations to be adaptive, the mechanisms that produce them must have certain properties. For the purposes of this discussion I will take an unabashedly adaptationist perspective and discuss the necessary design features of an adaptive-variation mechanism. This discussion does not require, or contain the assumption, that all intraspecific social system variation is adaptive (and reasons for expecting nonadaptive variation will be discussed later). However, many known instances of intraspecific variation appear adaptive and adaptation is a proper focus for much of our discussion.

5.2   ANALYZING SOCIAL SYSTEM VARIATION MECHANISMS

The first step in the analysis of an intraspecific variation mechanism is to determine the underlying nature of the difference from the individual organism's point of view. Several examples of mating systems variations seem due to differences in the distribution of the individuals in the populations caused by simple ecological forces. Examples are found among tree dwelling lizards (Manzur & Fuentes, 1979) woodrats (Escherick, 1981) and coral reef damselfish (Fricke, 1980). (See chapters 2 and 4).

In some cases it is hard to determine if a change in behavioral predisposition is involved. Both reedbuck and white-tailed deer are in larger groups when their habitat is more open (Jungius, 1971; Hirth, 1977). Do the deer and reedbuck live solitarily in closed habitat because they prefer solitude or because maintaining a group is too difficult there?

Alternatively, some features of open habitat may change the predisposition of these animals to aggregate. An example would be increased anxiety. If this anxiety were reduced by proximity to a conspecific, such a change would increase the predisposition to aggregate. If this second alternative proved correct, another question would be raised: is the changed psychological state an automatically initiated property of the animal that will occur whenever the individual is in more open habitat, or does it depend on individual experience such as attacks by predators or development in a situation in which the developing individual is exposed to aggregations regularly?

5.3   CONCEPTUALIZING ASSESSMENT

When the changes in social behavior do not involve a change in behavioral phenotype, there seems no need to postulate assessment. But when a change in behavioral predisposition is involved, especially a change leading to an adaptive outcome, it seems essential to postulate an assessment step. For example, if open habitat merely facilitates the expression of a pre-existing tendency to form groups, there is no need to posit an assessment step to account for grouping. However, if the tendency to group changes in open habitat then we must posit an assessment process that guides this change in behavioral predisposition. Suggestive evidence for a change in the predisposition to group would be a gradual change in group size after introduction to the new habitat.

The assessment process must assess the circumstances in which a particular social system is operating. In addition, some process must compare the effectiveness of the current social system with the effectiveness of one or more alternatives. For example, in order to adopt the most adaptive strategy for resource competition, an animal that is currently territorial must compare the efficiency of alternatives such as dominance, despotism and dominion in the current context of the ecology, demography and competitive strategies of others. The assessment should include one's own strengths *vis-a-vis* one's competitors because the system will not be equally favorable to all. It must also include an assessment of whether one is better or worse off to be interacting differently than one's conspecifics. There is a great deal of assessing to do and the quantitative effects of many variables of several kinds must be taken into account. Faced with a similar task we would probably prefer to be aided by a computer that would help us weigh up the several cognitively generated options. However, animals are more likely to make their assessments by some simpler process or 'rules of thumb'.

Assessing the consequences of alternative behavior patterns is essential. The nature of this assessment will likely vary from outcome to outcome (Bateson, 1987). For example, alternative foraging strategies could be compared by trying both and comparing the amount of food obtained. However, feedback will be much slower when the alternatives are different mating systems. The same feedback might not be available for months, and it could take years to try more than one system and compare the outcomes. Perhaps the animal assesses how well the current system is working; alternatively the two assessments may somehow involve one another. To guide an adaptive change in behavior the assessment process must produce right answers at least often enough to justify its costs and the costs of change. It must extract real information from the world.

This information must be accessible to the individual animal. In some cases the information will possibly be available cognitively but in other cases it won't and the animal will operate by a 'built-in' rule of thumb. If the reaction to the different circumstances is 'built in' then the assessment would be a simple process in which all that is required of the animal is the recognition that circumstances have changed. In this case the recognition of the change in circumstances incorporates recognition of their adaptive significance. Alternatively, the animal might have to learn the significance of the circumstances. If the animal is attacked more often in open habitat and consequently becomes more likely to join conspecifics in the open, then the significance of the difference in habitat is developmentally acquired. The animal need not assess significance in terms of its direct reproductive success. It could use correlates of reproductive success such as degree of predator-stimulated anxiety.

5.4   SAMPLING FOR ASSESSMENT

Research on the assessment process must discover how the animal perceives and evaluates those features of its environment that make adaptive shifts in social systems possible. The animal must do this by processing impinging stimuli. The animal cannot process what it cannot detect. Also it must perceive selectively and at least *attend* primarily to stimuli encoding useful information. Two kinds of information are worth gathering. One is information about the current ecological and social circumstances that could act as determinants of adaptive variation; the second is information about the future status of these same circumstances. An adaptive choice concerning whether or not to defend a foraging territory is mostly a function of immediate social and ecological circumstances. An adaptive choice concerning whether or not to change to a different mating system in birds is mostly a function of what the ecological and social determinants will be at the critical point in the use of the social system adopted, e.g., during the development of the young.

Obviously the indicator for the animal must predict the state of important features of their environment when they act in the present to select a social system that will pay off in the future. But equally, the animal will be reacting to some index of current circumstances in selecting the social system that will pay now. Therefore, to understand the assessment process we must know not only which features of the environment are important to the animal, but which features of the environment it will use as indices of those important features.

The 'decision' to defend or not to defend a foraging territory could follow a simple assessment process. First the local population density of conspecifics must be assessed. That density is an objective fact which various census techniques will ascertain with varying degrees of accuracy. We may count the number of species-specific calls heard at a particular time and place; we may count the number of animals seen per unit time while doing a transect; we may count the number of animals passing a certain point per unit time, etc. (Schemnitz, 1980). An animal could use any or all of these indices, depending on its mental or behavioral processes. We need to discover which of them they respond to.

Certain experiences vary with patchiness and so might offer possible assessment mechanisms. Variation in travel speed or variation in distance between units of food is a potential source of information. An animal foraging in a non-patchy environment would encounter food every so many steps, wing-beats, etc. with a small variation around the mean. An animal foraging in a patchy environment would experience large variation between units of food per unit of travel as it first passed through areas of concentrated sources of food and then through areas where food was sparse. Similarly the animal would experience variation in schedules of reinforcement while foraging in patches compared to when foraging between patches.

5.5   DIRECT AND INDIRECT INDICES

Different kinds of stimuli correlate with population density and other ecological variables and can be used in different ways. The most direct correlate of any ecological variable is a sample of the thing itself. For example, the animal moves about its home range and encounters food. This provides a sample of the incidence of the food over the rest of the home range.

The abundance of conspecifics (and other species of interest, such as competitors and predators) may be estimated from samples of correlates of their presence. Some of these correlates, such as the territorial songs of birds or scent marks by mammals, are specifically designed to signal the presence of an animal. Others, such as food items partially or wholly consumed, tracks, or the evidence of predation (e.g., mouse pellets produced by owls) are not.

The least direct correlates of relevant variables are those that predict the state of things to come; for example, correlates of future food abundance. Suppose a bird is deciding whether or not to express the potential to become polygynous. Sometimes the best predictor of a thing's abundance in the future is its abundance at the present. Red grouse (*Lagopus lagopus scoticus*) eat heather. Heather is a perennial plant, and the abundance of heather at the beginning of the breeding season may be a good index of red grouse numbers throughout the season. However, the present abundance of some variables does not predict their future abundance. An animal heavily dependent on the seeds of annual plants might need to decide about being polygynous before the seeds are produced. Such an animal would need to use a correlate of future seed numbers. It would be still more difficult to predict the future abundance of insects that eat annual plant seeds.

The correlates of ecologically significant variables discussed so far vary greatly in the degree to which they can be used to predict the ecological variables, but they are all in some sense direct and logical correlates of those variables. In fact, most of them are in a direct causal chain linking the variable and the predictor together. However, some potential or exploited correlates may not be. Any correlate the animal can perceive and has been a correlate in the past may be useful. We can illustrate this with an example somewhat removed from social behavior. The primary physiological determinant of respiration rate in vertebrates is the level of carbon dioxide in the blood. This is a predictor of the physiologically significant level of oxygen in the blood because they are strongly correlated, but they are not causally connected.

5.6   DEVELOPMENTAL DETERMINANTS OF ASSESSMENT

Assessment might occur at various developmental stages. Some correlation is likely between the developmental stage at which assessment occurs and the stage at which it is optimal for the animal to commit itself to a particular style of interaction. The earliest stage at which assessment might occur is in genetic differences between populations. In this case the assessment mechanism is natural selection, and the differences in interaction observed are relatively fixed outcomes of the natural selection process. This form of assessment would be most favored when the relevant ecological variables differ consistently for two populations or it is best to commit to a particular style very early. Perhaps the style in question is hard to acquire in later developmental stages, or there is little opportunity to assess the relevant variables in ecological time because the interactive style must be set before the variables are exposed to assessment. A possible example would be a population of birds that must nest colonially or solitarily. Suppose their breeding area has an annual influx of migratory nest predators during the egg stage of the birds. That source of predator pressure might vary from year to year, but the birds would have established their nests before they could assess the current year's level.

The second developmental point at which assessment might occur is in an early sensitive period (Caro & Bateson, 1986). This would be the optimal stage for assessment if the change in behavior can take place only at this stage, or if the critical information is most fully revealed at this time.

Another stage at which assessment might occur is at the beginning of some ecologically coherent unit of time. An example would be an animal that has seasonal breeding and whether or not it chooses to be territorial or colonial during this period. The abundance and distribution of food or the degree and kind of predator pressure experienced at the beginning of a season should determine this choice. The lemming population at the beginning of the breeding season of a kleptoparasitic jaeger accurately predicts the lemming population throughout the breeding season. Consequently, the mechanism which assesses that resource should operate each year at the beginning of the jaeger's breeding season. Therefore, the optimal assessment mechanism would assess at the beginning of each season and return to neutral between seasons. The jaegers could assess prey encounter per unit time, lemming vocalizations per minute, lemmings behaving aberrantly, ages of prey encountered, etc.

The present moment is still another developmental stage at which assessment might occur. Such a schedule requires that the ecologically relevant variables must be revealed by a correlate that expresses their distribution and abundance at the present time, and that changes in the present can produce an adaptive outcome. A foraging territory can depend on such a moment-to-moment assessment. Gill & Wolf (1975) have shown that golden-winged sunbirds shift adaptively between holding and abandoning territoriality as the level of nectar varies. Nectar production varies from season to season, from day to day and even from hour to hour within a day. Therefore, the sunbirds must monitor correlates of nectar level that vary from minute to minute.

5.7 PROCESSES THAT COULD PRODUCE ALTERNATIVE SOCIAL SYSTEMS

5.7.1 Choice

Whatever process assesses the level of nectar must be followed by one that produces a change in social interaction. This can happen only if the species or population has the potential for behavioral flexibility. To conceptualize the whole process clearly we must recognize a pivotal step in which the animal 'chooses' the system it will change to. This would be most clearly a distinctive step when the sequence of assessment, choice and change was managed in a highly cognitive way. The individual would 'know' its circumstances via assessment, 'know' the social system it was currently part of and/or the alternatives available to it, 'choose' one of those alternatives and 'change' social systems by changing behavior.

While this step is important conceptually, many change mechanisms are likely to be produced directly by assessment or guided strongly by change processes that develop directly from assessment (e.g., nutrition, hormonal changes, operant or classical conditioning, etc.). One of the features that distinguishes choice from change is that in choice the assessment process has to have the effect of predicting what others will do, at least if it is always to approximate optimal outcomes, while in change there is an established pattern both in the individual and in the other conspecifics to be assessed. Predicting the future behavior of others seems, at least on the face of it, a formidable challenge.

5.7.2. Change

Change must occur via one or more mechanisms. Change producing mechanisms must have a set of properties, which we will now consider. One major difference among the forms of intraspecific variation is the time course of the changes. In some cases generation after generation of different populations may manifest different social systems. So far as we know, hyenas in Ngorongoro, Tanzania, always live in territorial clans while those on the Serengeti, Tanzania, seldom do. Whatever mechanism accounts for this difference need not produce a change within the life of an individual. Each social system could be largely genetically fixed. In other cases the social system changes from year to year (e.g., California quail, Francis, 1965; McMillan, 1964). One or more proximate mechanisms must operate to make the individual behave one way in one year and differently in another year. In still other cases the social system changes from day to day or even from hour to hour (e.g., sunbirds, Wolf, 1978). (The mechanism producing this shift may work in minutes.)

5.8   GENETIC MECHANISMS

Intraspecific variation in social systems, like all biological phenomena, rests in some sense on genetically determined properties selected by natural selection. Consequently, a basic question about the mechanisms that produce such variation is: 'what has selection selected?' One set of properties that might have been selected are predispositions (Mason, 1979). For the present purposes it is useful to think of predispositions as tendencies to interact in particular ways, e.g., to be aggressive without site specificity as opposed to being aggressive only in a particular area. This definition must include their varying strength, their degree of robustness in the face of environmental variation, and experiences or nutritional states influencing their expression.

Animals can be genetically predisposed to interact in particular ways, as Seghers (1974) showed in guppies (see chapter 2). Taylor (1988) has shown that laboratory hatched and reared chinook salmon from populations that spawn near the ocean are less aggressive than those from populations that spawn further from the ocean. Taylor proposed that since aggression tends to produce territoriality in this species, selection has produced reduced aggression to facilitate earlier migration to the ocean in schools. Part of the strength of these demonstrations is that the differences were shown in the laboratory; field data alone cannot demonstrate genetic influences. Evidence that different behavior is manifested by genetically isolated populations does not prove the behavioral difference is genetic. Different populations could have the same genetic predispositions, but their expression could be modified by different circumstances. In fact, we know that some male cheetahs (*Acinonyx jubatus*) within a single population are social, defending a territory with one or more partners, while others remain solitary (Caro & Collins, 1987). These different phenotypes apparently have identical genotypes (O'Brien *et al.*, 1983).

Natural selection as a mechanism presents a somewhat different analytical problem than other mechanisms because it is no longer appropriate to distinguish between assessment processes and processes of change. At an earlier time in the history of these social system alternatives there may have been a process of assessment, but when change occurs through natural selection the assessment process at the individual level is lost in the selection history of the species. Alternatively one could think of assessment as taking place at the level of the population and thus retain the concept of assessment, but that is assessment in a different sense.

This mechanism would operate slowly and limit phenotypic flexibility, but it has advantages. It avoids the costs involved in phenotypic flexibility mechanisms (see chapter 7) and it can respond to ecological variables that are difficult to assess phenotypically.

Genetic differences alone cannot account for social plasticity that occurs within the individual in different circumstances or at different times, rather than between individuals (e.g., sunbirds). Selection for a particular degree of robustness in the predisposition to interact in particular ways also selects a degree of flexibility in that trait. Thus selection may have favored various degrees of sensitivity and responsiveness to social or ecological circumstances that would favor being predisposed to interact in particular ways.

5.9   EXPERIENCE MECHANISMS

Experience is a potentially powerful source of change that so far has seldom been shown to produce social system variation. Experience may alter behavior in many ways, and a large body of knowledge describes the impact of experience on behavior. However, little of that research has focused on changes in social interactions.

Generally speaking, the older tradition of learning assumed that all learning of responses followed a few simple paradigms. These paradigms could be studied in any one setting as effectively as in any other. The complexity of studying social interactions favored concentrating on simpler situations such as getting food or water or avoiding a standard negative stimulus such as an electric shock. It eventually became apparent that these paradigms did not account for all instances of modification of behavior by experience (e.g., Breland & Breland, 1967) and a recognition of species specificity and association specificity in learning is now well established (Garcia & Koelling, 1966; Bolles, 1975). However, the study of species specificity in the learning of social responses is not yet very far advanced.

One of the goals of the present review is to identify some of the aspects of behavior that studies of social learning should address. In a sense this will be a call for a broadening of the study of learning in an evolutionary-adaptive perspective to include study of the learning of social responses. However, it is also useful to consider the learning paradigms that have already been developed and explore their ability to account for some of the instances of intraspecific variation in social systems.

Potentially significant mechanisms include: habituation, sensitization, classical conditioning, instrumental conditioning, latent learning, observational learning, imprinting and similar sensitive-period effects, and cognition. We will probably not discover a reliable correlation between a particular social system outcome and a mechanism that produces it. In fact, several different mechanisms may produce the same outcome. However, each different mechanism may be revealed by the details of the interactions and the time course of the change. Therefore, it is critical to focus on the interactions, and not just their outcomes. The outcomes are important at the level of interaction with the ecology, but the mechanisms must alter interactions among individuals.

5.10 LEARNING THEORY AND SOCIAL SYSTEM PLASTICITY

Those of us concerned with the role of experience in the determination of social systems are consumers of learning theory rather than contributors to it. Learning theory has its own purpose and its own momentum. While its starting point is real world phenomena, the effort to analyze them rigorously and parsimoniously takes the form of developing hypotheses about the properties of animals and processes by which they relate to the real world, and then testing those hypotheses. The theorists are concerned primarily with increasingly closer scrutiny of their own and others' hypotheses.

We consumers want to make use of the properties and processes that are revealed in the course of theoretical work. They are potential explanatory tools that we can apply to the phenomena that interest us. We can hope to advance our understanding this way, and we must use this opportunity. However, there are no sure guidelines to success. The processes and properties that occupy the attention of theorists are studied, and often identified, in the laboratory. There they are isolated, by design, from the complexity of the real world that we are trying to understand. They should be relevant to that world, but there is simply no way to be sure if and how they are relevant in a particular case. Hence, there will be many missteps in their application to the social system phenomena we are trying to understand. We should not give up the attempt, but we must be cautious and prepared to be wrong sometimes (Mason, 1984).

5.11 LEARNING PARADIGMS

Learning theorists have established a number of paradigms via which experience modifies behavior. Perhaps the two most general are incorporated in stimulus–response (S–R) theory and cognitive processes theory. Because these two approaches seem so general, and because they often offer competing explanations for particular phenomena, I am discussing them at more length than some other processes by which experience may shape behavior.

S–R theory arises from the fact that certain pairings of stimuli and responses create new stimulus connections, e.g., classical and operant conditioning. The S–R paradigms are parsimonious and powerful. They keep us focused on the behavior itself (and hence on the immediate interplay between changes in circumstances and changes in behavior).

The direct shaping of behavior by contingencies is appealing. Finally, behavior often seems more habitual than rational, and S–R paradigms handle habits as well as, and sometimes better than, cognitive paradigms.

Nevertheless, there is plenty of evidence for cognitive processes as well. Animals are clearly capable of making and manipulating mental representations of their world (Mason, 1984, 1986; Dickinson, 1980; Terrace, 1984; Griffin, 1984). It would be hard to understand the behavior of free-ranging animals without supposing that they 'know' where the important features of their environment are. Many instances of assessment seem to require 'knowing' how abundant things are. Cognition is also attractive in its handling of apparent purposiveness or goal directedness of behavior (though not necessarily through knowing its consequences).

A cognitive approach seems particularly attractive to many of us concerned with social systems. The more radical cognitive position explains everything we see by analogy to a common-sense view of our own behavior when we are being rational, as we occasionally are. Yet accepting a radical cognitive position because we are immediately comfortable with it might serve us poorly. Group selection was once widely accepted for similar reasons, and it tended to obscure rather than highlight some of our best opportunities to understand animal social behavior. Besides, virtually all working cognitive psychologists suppose that the formation and manipulation of mental representations in animals cannot be more than roughly analogous to those processes in humans, where language provides such representational power.

5.12   AN ECLECTIC APPROACH

In the following pages I have drawn upon these and other paradigms of the effect of experience on behavior to suggest possible scenarios of assessment and change in social systems. In this chapter I have tried to set out the paradigms that might prove helpful in understanding social system variation and suggest some specific ways in which they might be useful. In chapter 6 I try to use these paradigms, along with other processes, to offer possible scenarios for assessment and change from one social system to another. I have done this eclecticly, sometimes mixing paradigms to account for a single social system event. For example, I might account for assessment via a cognitive process, then account for the change that follows in some other way, such as an S–R process or a sensitive period process.

We must not expect too much. Theoreticians developed most of these processes and properties to account for simpler transactions, e.g., an individual finding food. They may have difficulty accommodating the complexity of social interactions. However, the processes and properties are likely to have some useful generality, and we must explore their applicability to social system variation. As we do so we should also be aware of their deficiencies for our purposes, and make those explicit enough so the theorists can use our findings to refresh and refine their work.

We will probably be best served by a commitment to openness, and to a period of research in which the goal is to outline, then increasingly refine, our descriptions of the processes at work. Perhaps particular cases of intraspecific variation in social systems will stimulate study of processes involved in that particular case and reveal something general about learning.

5.13   SPECIFIC LEARNING MECHANISMS AND SOCIAL PLASTICITY

5.13.1   Classical conditioning

Classical conditioning is one potential mechanism. In the classical conditioning paradigm a stimulus comes to elicit a response formerly elicited only by a different stimulus. Pavlov's demonstration that a sound, after frequent pairing with meat powder, would come to elicit salivation in a dog is the prototypical example of classical conditioning. One way in which classical conditioning may account for intraspecific variation in social systems is if previously neutral stimuli come to elicit emotional responses which produce different social behavior, perhaps through acting as reinforcers in an operant paradigm.

If conspecifics can become conditional stimuli for emotional responses through being paired with unconditional stimuli for those emotional responses, this paradigm may be helpful in accounting for some instances of social system variation (Bolles, 1975). Consider the social system alternatives of living in a group or being solitary. If encounters with conspecifics regularly precede some fearful event, such as an encounter with a predator (which stimulates a fear response), the conspecifics might come to stimulate that response also, making them aversive stimuli and, hence, making the affected individual less social. Classical conditioning might also account for a shift from solitary to group living. If a predator or an aggressive conspecific repeatedly attacked a solitary individual but broke off the attack when the individual joined one or more conspecifics, then those conspecifics (or conspecifics in general) would be regularly associated with reduction of fear and might become anxiety reducing stimuli. In contrast, being alone would be associated with attacks and could become anxiety-producing.

I have now proposed two hypothetical histories: according to one, conditioning accounts for being solitary rather than being in a group. According to the other, conditioning accounts for being in a group rather than being solitary. The plausibility of each depends on predator behavior. If the predator seeks groups and ignores individuals, conditioned aversion to conspecifics might arise. On the other hand, if the predator is equally, or more likely, to attack solitary individuals, conditioned attraction might arise. Such plasticity on the part of prey would allow a single species to adjust to a rapid change in the strategy of a single predator or to a range in the relative abundance of different predators with different strategies. Prey species might be selected to condition toward one of the social alternatives more readily by the foraging predisposition of the predators of that species.

5.13.2 Operant conditioning

Operant conditioning persuasively accounts for changes in certain forms of behavior, e.g., locating food or shelter. There is a long tradition of creating potential models of operant conditioning (hypothetical histories of reinforcement) to explain particular social behavior patterns in humans (e.g., Skinner, 1938). We can imagine a plausible scenario by which a juvenile lizard learns to be territorial and expresses that territoriality when hungry. In this scenario the lizard attacks conspecifics within its home range and is almost immediately rewarded with access to a bit of food. Since the rate of a reinforced response goes up in the operant paradigm, the rate of attacking conspecifics within one's home range goes up.

5.13.3 Monitoring mechanisms

The adaptive value of the changes these mechanisms produce would be enhanced by a feedback mechanism that monitored the consequences of the changes and whether a change enhanced some correlate of fitness. Consequently, at least some monitoring mechanisms are likely. What might they be like? When intraspecific social system variation is produced by genetic differences, the monitoring mechanism is fitness manifested in direct or indirect reproductive success. This form of feedback provides an unambiguous evaluation of the value of the variation in behavior. However, selection will act on the overall value of the change mechanism, and so long as a particular mechanism is working better than any available alternative, it will be favored by selection, even though it does not always produce adaptation.

Feedback on the effect of intraspecific variation produced by classical conditioning appears likely to be limited to the persistence of the association between the unconditional and the conditional stimuli. The relationship persists only if they are paired at least occasionally (Bolles, 1975). This mechanism gives feedback in two forms. The first is feedback within the structure of the mechanism itself – in this case the reinforcement of the association – and the second is through selection on the value of having the mechanism, i.e., selection on the property of being conditionable.

Reinforcement following the response is the normal form of feedback from operantly conditioned behavior. In most cases the reinforcement would take a form such as food, water or sex. When the animal is motivated to have those, their occurrence following the response reinforces the response and assures its persistence. Again there is a second level of feedback in this case, in that selection has favored animals that are operantly conditionable by this reinforcement schedule. Recall the preceding hypothetical history of reinforcement by which a juvenile lizard is operantly conditioned to be territorial. A nice thing about this scenario is that the reinforcement would continue only so long as the animal was motivated by hunger and thus reinforced by food. When food became super-abundant two different things could happen: the animal might satiate its hunger and temporarily lose its aggressive motivation. Alternatively, a satiated animal's attack would no longer be reinforced by ingested food and so would undergo extinction.

This model might help us understand the social system variation observed in sunbirds. (It works best if home range loyalty is already built in.) It assumes that the animal is monitoring the behavior of conspecifics as a source of information about resources (Stamps, 1986), presumably via a cognitive process. It could begin with the animal attacking another that was eating. This requires only that the animal 'knows' it can get food where another individual is eating. A response learned by operant conditioning need not be reinforced every time it occurs, so the behavior could persist with attacks being reinforced only occasionally, so long as the subject was sufficiently hungry.

5.13.4   Secondary reinforcement

There is also a possibility of secondary reinforcement operating in this situation. A secondarily reinforcing stimulus takes on the properties of a primary (e.g., need-reducing) stimulus because of being paired with it. A conspecific retreating from attack might become such a secondary reinforcer. If it did, the subject would continue to defend its territory even when no longer hungry. By this scenario an animal could learn to defend a territory when hungry for a food reward, then continue to defend it when no longer hungry because of secondary reinforcement.

Several different behavioral properties could potentially produce defense of foraging territories. If the animal typically fed on non-renewable or very slowly renewable resources then its foraging strategy might be to defend its resources continuously. In that case selection might favor an animal in which territorial behavior was supported by secondary reinforcement and would continue to exclude conspecifics when it was not hungry. On the other hand, if the subject foraged on a transient or rapidly renewed resource, then its optimal strategy might be to defend resources when they are at a level where the benefits of defense exceed the costs and the subject is hungry, but not defend when the costs exceed the benefits, e.g., when there is plenty of food available and consequently the subject is no longer hungry. Shifts to and from foraging territories in both sunbirds (Gill & Wolf, 1975) and rainbow trout (*Salmo gairdneri*) (Jenkins, 1969) fit this model and might be explained by this mechanism. In the absence of secondary reinforcement, the exclusion behavior could decline either when it is rarely reinforced (little food), or when the subject is no longer hungry.

5.13.5   Cognition

Animals are able to construct and use something like mental representations of events in space and time and to establish causal connections between events (Dickinson, 1980; Mason, 1986). These properties are demonstrated by the animal's adaptive adjustments of their behavior that could not have been made without resort to such mental representations. Such representations must be developed by sampling, storing, and interpreting the individual's social and physical environment. Many of the assessment processes I have proposed incorporate such mental processes, and they seem essential. I make less use of cognitive processes in the change mechanisms I propose, but that may be due more to personal preference (or habit) than to any limitations in the potential of cognitive processes to produce social system change.

5.13.6 Habituation

Habituation might also produce intraspecific variation. In some species under some circumstances, this may result in a diminishing of territoriality. Habituation is a simple decline in responsivity to a stimulus which is not followed by any positive or negative consequences. When intruder pressure increases, the generalized stimulus of an intruder is presented at a higher rate. Habituation to such a stimulus might be favored in the phylogenetic history of some species because it would allow the animal to change adaptively when resource defense was no longer economically feasible. The following scenario illustrates this possibility.

We know that both intruder pressure and available resources can act as determinants of territoriality (see chapters 2 and 4). In some situations these two variables might be correlated. If intruder pressure increased because resources became more concentrated in the territory, the territory holder's assessment process would have made available the information that the additional benefits of having a territory would not justify the additional costs of defending it. However that assessment took place, it would not directly produce a change in the behavior: some other mechanisms would have to operate to produce change.

There could be an influx of intruders due to a migration or a catastrophic loss of immediately adjoining resources. In these cases the relaxation of territoriality would be unconfounded with increased resource abundance. It might be explained by either habituation or extinction of an operant response. An operant response could be extinguished as follows: the territory holder becomes territorial because when he attacks conspecifics he is reinforced by bits of food that the intruder has located within the territory holder's home range. If such attacks are thus reinforced within the area with which he is familiar (his home range) their frequency should increase and territorial defense will be the outcome. At moderate rates of intrusion, the defender may go on to the next attack quickly with no opportunity to eat the bit of food from which he has driven the intruder. Once established, operant responses can be maintained by only occasional reinforcement, so we could expect the behavior to be maintained. However, if the rate of intrusion by conspecific competitors becomes very high, the defender may go from one attack on a conspecific to another because there is nearly always another intruder in the area, requiring an immediate attack. In that case the schedule of reinforcement could become so lean that the behavior is extinguished.

A similar model could explain the relaxation of territoriality in individuals that have a superabundance of resources in their territory. If the individual is defending a territory in which superabundant resources develop, he is likely to be relatively satiated all the time. If satiated, the territory holder might be unlikely to eat the food after driving the intruder from it. If the pattern of driving conspecifics from the territory was developed in this individual via operant conditioning, the operant response would no longer be reinforced and could be expected to extinguish at some point. This model makes a specific prediction, incidentally, that territorial defense should wane gradually, even if food abundance increases suddenly.

5.13.7 Sensitive-period phenomena

Sensitive-period phenomena may explain some intraspecific variation. By sensitive-period phenomena I refer to some sort of developmental process that takes place over a short period of time and gives little or no further opportunity for flexibility in the individual's life. Several such recognized phenomena have varying degrees of potential to affect social interaction predispositions. Imprinting can have the effect of fixing the individual on one or another kind of object for particular forms of behavior: perhaps a similar process would fix an individual on certain patterns of behavior. Differences in early nutrition might predispose individuals to interact differently then and later. Exposure to hormones is often effective during a sensitive period.

The behavior of animals is more open to modification by experience at certain times than at others, and some of these periods of plasticity are critical to the kind of social relationships the animal forms and hence to the form of social systems toward which it is predisposed. For example, male red foxes tend to bond strongly with the first female with which they copulate, and remain monogamous. This makes the occasional occurrence of several pregnant females within the territory of a single male red fox anomalous (MacDonald, 1981; von Schantz, 1981; Zabel & Taggart, 1989; see chapter 4). However, experience during a sensitive period may account for this occasional polygyny. Breeders have observed that if the male fox is separated quickly from the first female he has mated and then goes on to mate with several different females during brief cohabitations, he will thereafter breed promiscuously (Enders, 1945).

The occurrence of such a sequence in nature could account for instances of polygyny, while the absence of such a sequence could account for only one of a group of females ever being pregnant. Suppose a pair establishes a territory and breeds alone for one season. If they were then joined by, or retained, additional females the breeding system would be monogamous, perhaps with helpers. On the other hand, if a naive male joined a group of females in a territory and they all came into estrus at about the same time he might breed several in a few days. The male fox would then be likely to breed unselectively. Such a disposition, combined with the home-range faithfulness of adult foxes, would produce a polygynous system.

It is clear that the psychological property that has been selected in this species can have outcomes other than monogamy. This property provides a mechanism whereby local abundance of resources can affect the breeding system. If the red fox mating system change were to occur according to this scenario, the assessment process and the change process would be indistinguishable.

A development-specific paradigm operating at a different sensitive period has been proposed to account for behavioral differences within a litter of coyotes (Bekoff, 1978). It has been suggested that in each litter of pups there are two roles: alpha and nonalpha. Once dominance relationships are formed, the alpha undergoes a fundamentally different socialization. It is less successful at inviting play, and in its social isolation it develops a different pattern of behavior. For example, Bekoff hypothesized that the alpha pup is much more likely to disperse. An implication for social systems is that a territorial pack is less likely when more of the potential members are of low sociability and have a high dispersal potential. Since each litter produces one alpha individual, any ecological factor that reduced litter size would cause shifts in the proportion of individuals with the alpha personality in the population, which in turn might affect the social systems.

5.13.8   Demographic effects on development

Variations in demographic structure can also change social systems because different age and sex classes typically behave differently. In an expanding population with low mortality, the young develop in a social environment containing more and older kin compared to young developing in a stable or decreasing population (Altmann & Altmann, 1979).

In animals that live in reasonably small, stable social groups the processes of birth, death, immigration, etc., can produce groups that vary in size and composition. Differences in group composition can affect not

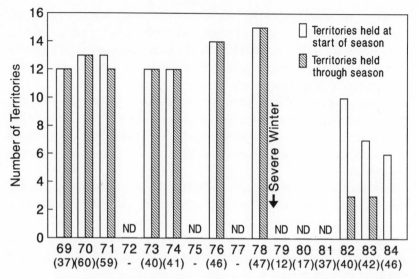

Fig. 5.1. Decline in territoriality in a pronghorn antelope population. The population was observed most years from 1969 through to 1984. The letters ND indicate years when presence or absence of territoriality was not recorded. The number of males present is indicated in parentheses below each year (data from Byers & Kitchen, 1988).

only the immediate group social system but also the developmental history of infants growing up in that group, and thereby influence their behavior as adults. The behavior patterns of the adults may influence subsequent generations, independently of demographic factors, and thus become a kind of 'cultural' determinant of that group's future social systems (Altmann & Altmann, 1979).

Byers & Kitchen (1988) attributed a shift in the spacing and mating system of an isolated population of pronghorns to a demographic change. For at least 15 years the females in this population were bred in territories held by a few older 'master' bucks (Bromley, 1969; Bromley & Kitchen, 1974; Kitchen, 1974). However, all the males over 4 and under 2 years of age died during the severe 1979 winter. Thereafter the territorial system gradually gave way to a non-territorial system (Fig. 5.1). Byers & Kitchen attributed the change to the lack of difference in territory holding ability among the remaining males. They said none were clearly superior enough to prevent the others from intruding. Consequently, intruders prevailed and first females, then males, abandoned the territories.

5.13.9 Imitation and culture

Culture is sometimes proposed to account for some instances of intraspecific variation in social systems (e.g., Bonner, 1980). This can be true if what one means by culture is the social processes that transmit behavior from one individual to another. The primary process used in cultural transmission among humans is language at a high level (Hill, 1978). That process is not applicable to other vertebrates. However, imitation or observational learning have been demonstrated in other animals. There are reported instances of the social transmission of some specific patterns of non-social behavior via observational learning (Mainardi, 1980), including sweet potato washing and panning for grain by Japanese macaques (*Macaca fuscata*) (Itani & Nishimura, 1973) and preference for particular foods by rats (Galef & Clark, 1971). Boyd & Richerson (1985) concluded that cultural transmission is rare in animals, and that when it occurs it affects a very narrow range of behavior.

Nishida (1987) reviewed evidence for imitation and cultural transmission of behavior in primates. He argued there is abundant evidence that primates learn from one another, but acknowledged it is nearly all field evidence and is, in effect, circumstantial. Galef (1988) reviewed the literature on imitation learning and concluded there is little experimental evidence that imitation *per se* actually occurs. He noted, however, that processes such as observational conditioning and social enhancement may support learning in social species. Unfortunately, these processes have come to light as alternative interpretations of data generated to demonstrate imitation in the strict sense. Therefore, these processes have not been developed in their own right, so their potential to influence social systems seems promising but remains unknown.

Consequently, on the one hand Nishida's 1987 and Bonner's 1980 suggestions that social patterns and social roles may be culturally transmitted provided a process that could account for cases of social system variation. Yet, on the other hand, rigorous demonstrations of such processes operating in animals are scarce and the precise paradigms by which they would operate are not known. Some important questions are yet to be addressed.

Before imitation, observational conditioning, or social enhancement can be used to account for social system variation the social transmission of social behavior must be demonstrated. Many asserted instances of imitative learning of non-social behavior have some overlap with ordinary operant conditioning. The subject's imitative act is rewarded, e.g., it gets food or water. Even poison avoidance is accomplished by imitating the food choices of the model, so this imitative act is physiologically reinforced by the ingested food. The imitation of social acts seldom leads to that kind of reinforcement.

Imitation in humans is often reinforced socially, for example, by approval. If such a process occurred in other animals, imitation learning might support the continuation of a particular spacing pattern. For example, if territorial signalling were imitated, territoriality could be transmitted from one generation to another. Young patas monkeys (*Erythrocebus patas*) have been observed to imitate the scent marking behavior of older group members (Hall & Goswell, 1964). If this occurred in the wild and a particular social system were produced by it, it would represent the social transmission of that social system.

Imitation or social facilitation of aggression has been demonstrated in some species. European blackbirds (*Turdus merula*) imitated conspecifics mobbing, even of as inappropriate an object as a plastic bottle (Curio, 1978). Male mice exposed to fighting as juveniles had shorter attack latencies and were more aggressive than males exposed to peaceful adults (De Ghett, 1975). Variation in the objects or intensity of social aggression could well influence the nature of the emergent social system.

5.13.10 Limitations of cultural processes

Such mechanisms would transmit the behavior pattern blindly, however, with no modification by feedback from the consequences of the behavior. Therefore behavior is less likely to vary adaptively. In this sense social reinforcement is fundamentally different from other kinds of reinforcement. When the reinforcement is food or water, the contribution of the behavior to physiological homeostasis is tested directly. Social feedback tests the homeostatic (biologically adaptive) value of behavior only indirectly, if at all. Of course, interacting socially in ways that produce successful relationships with social partners may well contribute to biological success. The process is still distinct, however, because the social patterns are reinforced by social rather than physiological reinforcers. Finally, before leaving the subject of imitation, we should note that while imitation could account for a social system's persistence or spread, it cannot account for its onset or termination.

In summary, then, imitation and cultural transmission may contribute to our understanding of intraspecific variation in social systems in the future, when (and if) these phenomena are firmly demonstrated and some details about when and how they can influence social behavior are known. Perhaps our increased awareness of social system variation will help to identify opportunities to study these processes and their consequences. But in their present state of development it is not obvious how to make use of them to account for particular instances of intraspecific variation in social systems.

5.14   HORMONAL AND METABOLIC FACTORS

5.14.1   Prenatal hormonal influences

One possible source of variation in social systems of adult mammals is the prenatal influence of various hormones. Rats born of mothers stressed during pregnancy are more anxious as adults. This could alter their later, adult social system by making them more prone to join conspecifics in anxiety-provoking situations, i.e., their greater anxiety might make the anxiety-reducing effect of proximity to conspecifics more reinforcing. This would influence the outcome of experiential effects on social behavior. For example, desert wood rats, *Neotoma lepida*, are often territorial where there are no avian predators (Vaughan & Schwartz, 1980, see chapter 2). The more anxiety an individual experiences, the more aversive leaving cover to defend territory would be. Consequently, one possible determinant of living in an undefended home range would be the endocrinological consequences of being born to a mother who had experienced the higher stress associated with higher predation pressures. This social system change could also affect the breeding system. Animals living in territories controlled by a single male are more likely to be monogamous or polygynous than to breed in other systems.

Stress experienced by the mother might also affect the parental care expressed by males. More anxious individuals might be more inclined to be reinforced by the presence of conspecifics. Some mice are known to show a two-parent parental system when in unusually dense aggregations (Mihok, 1979), presumably because the males are exposed to young and become parental through the process of 'sensitization' (Noirot, 1972). In some species communal, rather than one-parent or two-parent, systems could be produced by the same mechanism.

Testosterone production is altered in the male fetuses of female rats stressed during the last days of pregnancy (Ward & Weisz, 1980). The testosterone pulse comes earlier than usual, and the fetuses are not exposed to testosterone at the normal stage of prenatal development. Their nervous systems undergo less masculinization and defeminization than those of unstressed mothers. Such males show less sex-typical behavior as adults (Clemens & Glaude, 1978). This may have broad effects on their social behavior and consequently on the social system they produce. Various forms of aggressive behavior have been shown to be related to male testosterone level (Christie & Barfield, 1979), and the establishment of such reproductively oriented social systems as territoriality could be affected by this condition.

Female mice exposed to testosterone as fetuses behave differently as adults. Females positioned between male siblings inside the uterus are partially masculinized and defeminized (vom Saal & Bronson, 1980). As adults they are more aggressive, less attractive to males, and more inclined to urine mark their environment. All these behavioral differences seem likely to have social system consequences. This change can have a complicated history. In the first place it is due to the testosterone levels produced by their male siblings during intrauterine development. Since the testosterone level of these males can be determined by the stress to which their mothers are exposed, the adult phenotypes of female mice seem likely to be determined in part by their mother's exposure to stress.

This phenomenon could in turn act as a breeding system determinant. Armitage (1977, 1988) has concluded that the aggressiveness of the first female a particular male yellow-bellied marmot (*Marmota flaviventris*) mates with largely determines whether he is monogamous or polygynous. A single aggressive female that attacks all immigrant females will keep the territory free of other females and hence produce a monogamous breeding system. Less aggressive or more sociable females tolerate additional females in the territory and make polygyny possible. Armitage suggested that the phenotypic differences between female yellow-bellied marmots are genetically determined, but the aggressive phenotypes could be partially determined by their masculinization as fetuses.

5.14.2 Postnatal hormonal effects

Hormonal changes can also act in the present to produce changes in social systems. Wingfield *et al.* (1987) reported that monogamous species have high testosterone levels only early in the breeding season, while polygynous species have high testosterone for most of the breeding season (Fig. 5.2). Moreover, an individual pied flycatcher's testosterone level corresponds to his mating pattern. When they breed monogamously, they have the monogamous testosterone pattern and when they breed polygynously, the polygynous testosterone patterns. This work also reveals something about the process via which testosterone (or its metabolities) can influence behavior. At least some songbirds initiate territorial defense while their testosterone levels are low, but they will not continue to defend their territory unless the testosterone levels rise. Perhaps testosterone (or its metabolities) influences this behavior by preventing the territorial male from habituating to the intrusion of other males. Mays *et al.* (1989) found, surprisingly, that adult male Harris' hawk helpers had higher testosterone titers than breeding males.

5.14.3 Nutritional effects

Changes in the nutritional state of individuals can also have a significant effect on the social system they produce, in at least some cases through producing changes in those individuals' hormonal state.

The blood's protein level determines its testosterone carrying capacity (Lloyd & Weisz, 1975). Poor physical condition or poor diet could indirectly lower blood testosterone, thus possibly changing social behavior. With lower circulating testosterone, several reproductive social system changes could occur. Less aggressive males may be more likely to aggregate. In aggregations, males are more likely to be exposed to young and therefore, to become parental by 'sensitization' (Noirot, 1972). By this same mechanism, increased patchiness of food resources (which

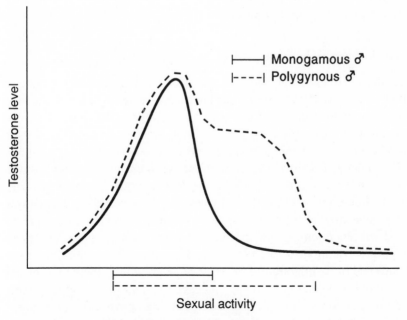

Fig. 5.2. Testosterone levels of monogamous and polygynous pied flycatchers (redrawn from Wingfield *et al.*, 1987).

might be produced by drought) could sharply increase the nutritional differences between males, and thus the blood's testosterone carrying capacity. Consequently, better-fed individuals could be more aggressive. Such an uneven distribution of aggressive behavior among the males could produce a shift from territoriality (often associated with monogamy) to despotism (which is almost always associated with polygyny).

Poorly nourished females frequently do not go through the endocrine changes associated with reproduction. If food were scarce and unevenly distributed (for example, because of dominance relations between females), the upshot would be that only some would reproduce. Some of those that did not might remain and function as helpers. This could produce a shift from a parental care system to a system of helpers at the nest (Lenington, 1980). On the other hand, well-nourished female birds might recover the endocrinological characteristics of breeders quickly after producing the first clutch. This potential for rapid clutch production might combine with an endocrinological state appropriate to initiating mating. That, in turn, might produce a shift from monogamy to serial or even simultaneous polyandry in exceptionally well nourished females.

As we have already noted, a shift in one social system may produce change in another. In these cases, shifts from monogamy to either polygyny or polyandry are likely to be accompanied by shifts from two-parent care to one-parent care.

5.14.4   Ingested hormone effects

In addition to general nutritional effects on the endocrinological state of females, ingested hormones could have a marked effect on reproductive social behavior. Gonadotropic hormone production has been shown to be modified in several herbivorous vertebrates by the contents of their food plants. Green plants enhance reproduction in some rodents, rabbits (Friedman & Friedman, 1939; Bradbury & White, 1954), and possibly white crowned sparrows (*Zonotrichia leucophyrys*) (Ettinger & King, 1981), but inhibit reproduction in voles (Berger *et al.*, 1977). High levels of phytoestrogens in the plants eaten by sheep severely disrupt reproductive functioning, but specific behavior changes have not been reported (Bennets *et al.*, 1946; Adams *et al.*, 1981). California quail reproduction is inhibited in years of poor growth of their food plants (Leopold, 1977). Some evidence suggests the inhibition of at least their egg production is due to plant foods with high phytoestrogen concentrations in drought years (Leopold *et al.*, 1976). Male Japanese quail (*Coturnix coturnix*) fed biochanin A, an important phytoestrogen, show sharply decreased levels of courtship and copulatory behavior (DeMan & Peeke, 1982). In species in which these behavior patterns are important for pair-bonding, their absence might produce a general breeding failure or a shift from monogamy to promiscuity. DeMan & Peake (1982) did not observe any reduction in the number of eggs produced by treated subjects. In this experimental setting (a male and a female together in a small cage) mating system effects could not have been seen.

5.14.5   Social-experience effects on behavior-determining hormones

Stress experienced as an adult, such as losing a fight, can reduce testosterone levels (Rose *et al.*, 1971). During periods of social instability or reorganization the subordinate males have substantially lower testosterone levels (Sapolsky, 1987). There are several situations in which the number of fights lost differs in different social systems. Topi in an all-purpose territory have many fewer border encounters than topi in a lek (Monfort-Brahm, 1975). Each rebuffed attempt to cross a border is a loss. Therefore, lekking topi have more losses and tolerate much closer neighbors, at least after the system has matured. It is a long leap to suggest that topi are less aggressive because their losses have reduced their testosterone and hence testosterone-motivated aggression. But some mechanism is clearly operating, and some such hypothesis is necessary.

A shift in reproductively oriented social systems might also occur when crowding at a resource creates a situation in which normally territorial animals must aggregate. When that happens some individuals will lose many fights to the dominant individual. Under these circumstances a despotism system tends to develop (e.g., Evans, 1951; Berry, 1974). Lower-level individuals would be likely to produce much less testosterone. This can set up a shift from a breeding system of territorial monogamy to aggregated polygyny.

I have proposed some speculative answers to some of the questions raised by intraspecific variation in social systems. I hope I have identified some fruitful research possibilities. I am certain I have shown social system variation raises a rich set of questions.

6

Social system variation
mechanisms: products

The conceptual review of proximate processes in chapter 5 has laid the background for this chapter. Here we will consider particular examples of social system variations and develop hypotheses about the proximate mechanisms that might have functioned as both the assessment and change processes, then review some possible strategies for research on such processes.

6.1   SOLITARY AS AN ALTERNATIVE TO GROUP

6.1.1   Predation

Predation may determine group versus solitary living via several different mechanisms. In the guppies Seghers (1974) studied, one population consistently grouped and another was consistently solitary. This difference proved to be heritable. We can explain this intraspecific difference as we explain interspecific differences in traditional socioecology, i.e., we invoke natural selection. For these purposes, natural selection becomes the mechanistic explanation for the observed differences in social behavior. In fact, the demonstration that the predisposition was inherited makes the evidence that natural selection produced this social system variation stronger than in many cases of interspecific differences.

Predation might produce social system change through other means as well. When animals live both in groups and solitarily in the same population, the assessment and change mechanisms probably operate in ecological time manifesting plasticity built into the whole population. In these cases they will be separate processes that we may be able to analyze individually.

In chapter 5 I proposed that for individuals which got relief from predator attack in the presence of conspecifics, the conspecifics would become, in effect, safety signals, increasing their attractiveness. In this model the experience of the predator attack would be the material for the assessment process and sustained predator-associated anxiety would be the assessment process itself. The change process would be a learned or unlearned response to the predator-associated anxiety by a reduction of that anxiety in the presence of conspecifics. In that case the conspecifics would have become safety signals and hence, attractive (Dickinson, 1980).

This model will work only if the animal is not averted by observing a successful predator attack on another group member (the larger the group the more likely that is). A species can be subject to such aversion. When pen reared wild turkeys (*Meleagris gallopavo*) were released into the wild, each rearing group assembled every night to roost. However, when a predator killed one of the flock it disbanded and never again reassembled (Leopold, 1944). In this example the assessing animal must have responded directly to experiencing a successful predator attack on a flock member. The assessing animal would also be more anxious while roosting in a group. In this case roosting solitarily would be less anxiety provoking. This decrease in anxiety while alone would reinforce the behavior of roosting alone and would act as the change process in this social behavior shift. Such a predisposition might select for predators that find groups more readily than solitary individuals. A predator that searched by monitoring prey social interactions would tend to find groups. Species that flock more under more predator pressure must be predisposed to respond differently to such an experience.

It is also possible, and perhaps more likely, that in many species conspecifics are already anxiety reducing. In that case variations in degree and consistency of predator produced anxiety would account for solitary and group living as alternative patterns. The impact of predation on sociality in most species will probably be to bring individuals together into groups (though the turkeys illustrate the possibility for the opposite effect). However, individuals in groups will often experience greater competition for resources like food or water. In such circumstances a shift to a solitary pattern would increase each individual's success in obtaining such resources. The proximate mechanisms producing a change from group to solitary living present an interesting conceptual challenge. Seghers (1981) suggested hunger and anxiety may act as opposite vectors so that an individual spot shiner (*Notropis hudsonius*) may become solitary when hunger overrides the anxiety it experiences when solitary, then join a group when it has eaten. According to this hypothesis this variation in social systems is in response to predation, but predation as such is not assessed; instead the degree of need for food is. The anxiety stimulated by predators is assumed to remain constant while need for food varies. Such a process would be optimal under constant levels of predation. Of course, it might not be optimal but merely an available strategy that is better than no plasticity at all.

6.1.2   Forced aggregation

Another developmental hypothesis is circumstances that force animals to be together will increase their predisposition to form groups. African jewel fish (*Hemichromis bimaculatus* Gill) live in freshwater in areas where the volume of water is occasionally reduced by drought. They usually school until about 100 days old, then disperse and set up territories. But when they are crowded during development, they continue to school until at least 160 days old (Coss & Burgess, 1981). In uncrowded jewel fish the number of dendritic spines on tectal interneurons increased between 100 and 160 days, when they reached the adult level. But the number of dendritic spines did not increase in the crowded juveniles (Burgess & Coss, 1981). This suggests a possible neural basis for this social system alternative.

Gilbert (1978) found that group-reared axis deer (*Axis axis*) were more social as adults, and Hirth (1977) suggested the association of white-tailed deer females in open habitat caused their young to develop in a more social atmosphere and so to be predisposed to be more social as adults. (Perhaps conspecifics could become secondary reinforcers by being paired in the individual's experience with nursing and foraging.) Hirth's suggestion may not explain his white-tailed deer data. One group of captive-reared white-tailed deer were not more social after higher density rearing (Collias, 1950). Still, this paradigm may well explain some instances of these social systems being expressed as alternatives.

An interesting feature of Hirth's hypothesis is that the assumed value of the grouping is to reduce predation by the wolf, a predator no longer present in either of the ecosystems studied (but coyotes are still present in both). In this case the assessment process would be vulnerability experienced over one time scale (evolutionary) perceived over another (ecological). That is also true of the shiner example above, but the shiner varies in behavior from moment to moment, while the white-tailed deer appears to be stable during and across generations. According to this hypothesis the assessment of vulnerability has remained constant despite not being reinforced through experiencing predation. Note that the hypothetical mechanism is not directly related to the proposed function of group formation.

6.1.3   Increased resource availability via group membership

Barlow (1974) reported that territory holding competitors attack each solitarily foraging manini much more often than each member of a feeding school in the same area. Attacked manini shift from foraging solitarily to foraging in schools. The school dilutes the territory holders' defense so members of schools feed at a higher rate.

Barlow (pers. comm.) has suggested an interesting potential mechanism to account for the observed shift. He proposed manini always tend to join conspecifics they encounter high in the water column. Attacks by territorial food competitors send them high into the water column where they encounter conspecifics more often. Thus the groups are an essentially automatic outcome of the combination of that predisposition and their displacement.

When we analyze this hypothesis in terms of assessment and change processes, the assessment process appears to consist of the rate at which the individual experiences attacks or threats that moves it up in the water column. This hypothesis does not posit the operation of any intervening variables or any internal change in the manini. The change process consists entirely of the unmodified operation of the predisposition to approach other manini that are up in the water column at the same time.

However, the same data could be accounted for by an hypothesis using intervening variables, and such an hypothesis offers an instructive contrast at this point. The contrast begins with the assessment process. According to the intervening variable hypothesis the attacks not only change the immediate behavior of the attacked individual, but also produce a longer term internal change of increased anxiety which is the key assessment factor. The anxious manini change because their anxiety is reduced when conspecifics are present. The hypothesis assumes that because of individual or selective history, conspecifics are more attractive when manini are anxious. Anxious manini approaching conspecifics form schools.

It may be possible to test these alternative hypotheses by finding a way to move manini into the water column without their being threatening or attacked. A cue as to whether or not attack initiates some internal process would be whether or not their flight distance or time up in the water column increased. Another interesting index would be their latency to leave the school.

Social systems also vary when a member of a group has access to food unavailable to a solitary individual. Coyotes vary from solitary to group living. Group living coyotes are often feeding on the carrion of large mammals or even capturing large mammals (Bekoff & Wells, 1980; Camenzind, 1978; Bowen, 1981). Solitary individuals could form groups as follows: a mated pair is the basic reproductive unit. Both parents feed the young, in part by regurgitating food at the den. When the young are older they accompany the parents. In a habitat (community) with a number of large mammals, carrion would be an important source of food. Access to, and possession of, carrion would be enhanced by being in the company of pack members who would help the individual compete with other scavengers. Under these conditions families are known to form stable packs that last for generations (Bekoff & Wells, 1980).

In this case the assessment process might consist of a reaction to the degree of hunger experienced under different circumstances. A solitary animal would be no more likely to find carrion than a member of a group, and would be much less likely to be able to defend it. Consequently it will be hungrier when alone than when with other members of its pack. The change process might be very closely linked with the assessment process. While the assessment process takes place the other members of the pack gradually become discriminative stimuli for hunger reduction. Consequently, they would attract one another. Eventually they could take on some sort of secondarily reinforcing properties and being close could become an end in itself. To avoid aggression the individual would draw upon its repertoire of friendly or ingratiating behavior.

6.2   COLONIALITY AS AN ALTERNATIVE TO TERRITORIALITY

6.2.1   Assessment via learning

Territoriality frequently alternates with coloniality in some birds (see chapter 2). Each alternative can be an adaptive adjustment to the distribution of suitable nest sites, if the assessment process achieves a weighted comparison of the suitability of nest sites and the proximity of neighbors. Such an assessment must include evaluation of nest sites. Experienced breeders have several possible ways to assess nest sites. The first is that they may have attempted to breed at this site in the past. If the breeding attempt was successful, they might be more likely to breed there again. Experienced breeders also might generalize from their success in attempted breeding at a similar site in the past.

Inexperienced breeders might assess a nest site in several ways. One source of information is the birds' experiences outside of the breeding season. Many raptors prefer high perches that give a good view of the surrounding area, and many choose such sites for nests. In this case the site's suitability for nesting could be assessed by its suitability for perching. In other cases the inexperienced bird may have a 'build-in' shift to a nest site preference under the influence of reproductive hormones. Animals that produce burrows or dens for their young by digging may experience the development of a preference for a particularly suitable soil. Suitability could be assessed by brief digging bouts. Other preference shifts could guide assessment of other areas in similar ways (e.g., a shift to a preference for noisy neighbors).

6.2.2 Change from territoriality to coloniality via experience

Breeding experience

After assessment has been completed the individuals will need either to select a system (if they are not participating in one) or change systems (if they are participating in a particular one). The social system outcome following this assessment will depend on the animal's predispositions. The animal may be predisposed to be distant from neighbors but accept coloniality in order to have a better nest site than it can find in isolation. On the other hand it may prefer to be close to neighbors but accept distance in order to get a desired nest site.

This distinction has an additional wrinkle in breeding systems; seasonal breeders must make a selection at the beginning of each season. Selection might follow directly from assessment: if the animals try building a nest at various sites and settle at the best, nest site selection will have determined their spacing system. On the other hand, the selection process may consist of a developmental history. For example, in some species individuals that spend more time in an area defend it more (Wiley & Wiley, 1980b).

Food distribution

Food supplies that cannot be predicted in space may produce selection of the spacing system by creating disparity between the amount of time spent in feeding locations and nest sites. An animal feeding on a spatially unstable food supply may spend too little time in any one area to begin to defend that area, while spending plenty of time at the nest site to begin defending it. The same animal feeding on a stable food supply surrounding the nest site might spend enough time in both to become defensive about both. Time alone could produce these effects only in an animal predisposed to become defensive of the familiar.

Osprey might select coloniality rather than territoriality by a different mechanism. The mechanism might involve the birds using one another as a source of information about food (Greene, 1987). They might approach each other nonthreateningly to avoid driving off an approaching source of information. The information obtained (and cognitively represented) could reinforce such approaches. Thus exploiting one another for information could produce a pattern of amicable interaction, and even make each other's presence secondarily reinforcing. With the onset of the breeding season the neighboring perches could become nest sites, and the outcome would be a colony.

A related but slightly different selection process would consist in the animal becoming colonial by settling on a suitable nest site and beginning to forage from this site. If sources of food are near the nest the individual may find itself competing directly with others for food. The sites of victories in aggressive competition over a food item may come to be defended (the lizard data suggest this). If the food resources are consistently located near the nest site, the individuals may build up a set of victory sites or sources of food visible from the nest. If the sight of a conspecific stimulates it to go and compete for food whenever a conspecific seems to be foraging successfully and the sources of food are distributed near its perch the area will function as an all-purpose territory.

Predation

Predator pressure also determines alternation between coloniality and territoriality. Assessment of predator pressure might take many forms, including the following scenario. Suppose that the prey species has a well-established stimulus-pattern-recognition that translates to predator. It could be sight, sound, smell of the predator's scent posts, etc. If these stimuli consistently make the prey anxious, that anxiety could act as an assessment process. Such assessment could lead to system selection in at least two ways. The first supposes that individuals are pre-programmed to find both predators and conspecifics aversive and that the intensity of each aversion is a function of their proximity to the relevant stimulus. If being closer to a conspecific reduces predator stimulated anxiety, then the higher the predator aversion (stimulated by predator sightings, etc.) the closer to conspecifics will the two avoidance gradients meet. When the result is that the individuals are very close to their conspecifics before the gradients meet, they are colonially organized.

6.2.3 Change via development

A system selection mechanism that might operate more remotely in time is the effect of a pregnant mother's stress on the later behavior of her offspring. The more anxious offspring respond more to predators and thus are predisposed to coloniality. This mechanism could explain the difference in territoriality between wood rat populations. Nonterritorial behavior could be transmitted generation after generation from anxious mothers to yet unborn sons, and maybe even predispose daughters to produce such sons in the next generation. Distinguishing genetic differences from such an environmental mechanism would be a nice research problem.

6.2.4 Change via selection

Of course, change from territorial to colonial systems could take place in evolutionary time with natural selection driven by predation acting as the mechanism. Suppose that a territorial pattern is already established, and in the current circumstances produces more fitness than a colonial pattern. Then a new predator arrives whose style makes colonial individuals much more successful than territorial. Natural selection, by favoring genetic predispositions to be closer, would select for colonially predisposed individuals, and hence a colonial population.

A change occurring in ecological time might also be produced by predation on animals selected to be plastic. Suppose a population is breeding territorially and becomes subject to a predator that can overcome a solitary pair's defense but can be mobbed by several birds. If a pair were to lose its eggs early in the nesting season it could be predisposed (through selection) to relocate before laying again. The predator might have two effects: to make the birds less inclined toward conspicuous territory defending displays and to make them more anxious. If mobbing were reinforcing, spending time near conspecifics would become reinforcing since it would be the setting for experiencing mobbing. This shift could also be produced by predation in other ways. If predator pressure on solitary individuals were high before the breeding season they might tend to feed in flocks and roost communally. With the onset of the breeding season their predator maintained gregariousness could lead them to settle near one another and thus be colonial.

6.3   TERRITORIALITY AS AN ALTERNATIVE TO COLONIALITY OR DOMINANCE

6.3.1   Changing from colonies to territories

There are several ways in which a shift from a colonial to a territorial system might occur. Colonial birds are often central place foragers. Central place foraging (travelling from a central place such as a roost, nest site or burrow to forage elsewhere, then returning to the nest site) requires more travel (Hamilton & Watt, 1970). Anything that increased the cost of travel or decreased the benefits of co-location could tilt the balance of benefits toward territoriality (see chapter 2). Suppose the forage resource becomes increasingly patchy or increasingly stable in space. An individual might begin to commute regularly from a colony site to a particular foraging area and begin to defend it and roost there. Roosting there would increase its familiarity with the area and increase its chances of nesting there. This could be reinforced if females were more inclined to settle in a space with abundant food.

6.3.2   Assessment preceding dominance replacing territoriality

In at least some of the mechanistic processes that produce this outcome the first step must be assessment. Variation in the hippo social systems described in chapter 2 (Karstad & Hudson, 1986) illustrate these concepts. Male hippos on the Mara River in Kenya were territorial when the water was high and pools abundant. This strictly territorial system shifted to a dominance system when many of the pools became too small for the hippos. First the females and then the males left those pools and went to the still filled pools, joining the territorial male and the resident females. There the new males behaved as subordinates.

The males in the diminishing pools experienced these ecological changes via several sensory channels. They would experience drier skin in various ways. They might also experience more airborne insects. Their body and skin temperatures would rise if the water no longer covered them. They might get sunburned. The consequences of hippo occupation, such as hippo dung, would become increasingly concentrated in the shrinking pool, at least until the females left. Once the females left, the males would experience their absence. Any and all of these sensory and social experiences could serve as assessment mechanisms.

We could imagine these sensory inputs affecting the hippo's behavior either via some cognitive process or via an S–R response paradigm. An

S–R paradigm could work by assuming these stimuli were noxious and the animal had a history of escaping them by going to another pool. A cognitive scenario could work by assuming that some of these stimuli had been followed by greater discomfort in the past, and this relationship was encoded in a mental representation of the subject's history. While the next step in the process, knowing the location of the next pool, could be handled by either approach, the cognitive approach of assuming some sort of mental representation of the location of the pools seems most parsimonious.

The behavior of these hippos is unlikely to change gradually, with intermediate points. When a male leaves one pool he must soon enter another and must quickly change to a social behavior pattern that makes it possible for him to stay there. These two changes are probably due to two separate processes: one that changes location and the other that changes behavior pattern. The change of location requires processing of information and the coherent use of it. Here the assessment step is distinct and unique.

After changing location the hippo changes his behavior. He becomes subordinate by activating an alternative interactive style. This works, because the territory holder also activates an alternative interaction style; he dominates, but no longer excludes, a rival who behaves subordinately (Rodman, pers. comm.). Somehow each hippo taps his alternative repertoire.

6.3.3   Assessment combined with change

In other cases the assessment step may not occur separately but be built into (or precluded by) the mechanism that determines the interaction pattern. For example, in some species the development of site defense that defines territoriality depends on spending a certain amount of time at a particular place (Wiley & Wiley, 1980a,b). When food is evenly but sparsely distributed the animal may not spend enough time in any one place to become defensive of it. The lack of territoriality in pronghorn populations living in low productivity habitat may have been produced by this process. Similarly, pronghorns abandoned territories in productive habitat when hunting pressures frequently displaced territorial males (Copeland, 1980). Reduction in site-occupancy time may have caused this abandonment.

The golden-winged sunbird's hour to hour shift of spacing systems from territoriality to dominance, according to the economics of territorial defense, provides another opportunity to conceptualize these processes.

Apparently these birds start fresh every morning, selecting a behavior pattern at the beginning of each day, and then perhaps changing when the payoff changes. The assessment process might take several forms. It could use the ratio of flight time to feeding time, or a derived index such as whether the individual is experiencing a net loss or net gain in energy. Alternatively it could use the direct sensory experience of drinking from flowers. It experiences both the concentration and volume of sugar in the nectar and could estimate the value of the average flower from the value of the flowers sampled, or it could monitor the volume of nectar ingested per unit of time regardless of the number of flowers visited.

6.4   TERRITORIALITY AND LEKKING AS ALTERNATIVES

6.4.1   Developmental mechanisms

Territoriality could supplant lekking via a developmental mechanism. Suppose lekking was produced proximately in a dense population via the intensity of intruder pressure on individual territory holders. If a lekking population experienced a substantial decrease, territory holders would experience a lower encounter rate. This would enable them to defend females over a larger area. These larger areas could come to include foraging resources as well as a breeding arena and eventually be classified as territories. (Note that this scenario would be most readily revealed via a descriptive system in which gradients are described rather than dichotomies.) This change scenario depends on a particular lek-development scenario. In fact, leks could be determined in a number of ways, and a shift to territory in as many or more ways.

A lekking system could be changed to territoriality by natural selection. The following is a plausible hypothetical history: lekking has developed as a consequence of hot spots – areas where females are concentrated by the presence of some sort of resource (Bradbury & Gibson, 1983; Clutton-Brock, 1990). Consider the topi example described in chapter 4, in which the resource is the lower level of nocturnal predation on open meadows. Now suppose that the incidence of predation by lions drops precipitously. The balance of costs and benefits shifts so the females do better if they avoid the lekking area (e.g., they are harassed less by breeding males). Natural selection would begin to favor a female preference for males away from the lekking area, favoring territorial males.

We can also imagine this shift taking place developmentally. Let us assume the lekking system is due to the density of the population manifested as intruder pressure on the size of the defensible area. A reduction in the intruder pressure would allow the size of the defended space to expand. An expanded defended space could eventually include enough resources to cross the categorical threshold from lek to territory.

Change might or might not be preceded by such a separate assessment step. For example, the assessment process might not involve any transduction of information about the environment but be an internal process in which changes in blood chemistry cross a threshold so behavior patterns shift or change in frequency. In that case assessment would be through a physiological change rather than a perceptual change. Perhaps some short term correlate of nutritive state, such as blood sugar level, acts directly on some component of aggressivity that produces change from site defense to status defense.

Development under conditions of poor nutrition might produce territoriality as an alternative to dominance. In some species poor nutrition during development reduces play and increases aggressivity so that unforewarned and relatively ungraded aggression is the typical response to conflict (Frankova, 1973; Barres *et al.*, 1970). If a dominance system requires graded aggression, ungraded aggression seems more likely to produce a territorial system.

6.5   TERRITORIALITY AS AN ALTERNATIVE TO DESPOTISM

Whatever organismic or other variables determine whether the shift from territory is to dominance or despotism, a shift to despotism still requires the steps necessary to employ any alternative system. A possible assessment step is illustrated by the lizards that shift from territoriality to despotism (Berry, 1974). The lizards could have experienced decreased food internally, externally or both. Change could begin with the food deprived individuals moving toward detectable sources of food. The owners of those resources would probably have dominance advantages over all newcomers, while the newcomers would have none over each other, since none would be accustomed to winning in that space.

A long lasting mechanism might produce their subordinate behavior. Starved individuals might have low testosterone levels when they enter the territory. They might all behave subordinately, leaving the territorial individual as a tyrant. For the change to be completed the tyrant also has to stop chasing subordinates when he gets exclusive access to a particular source of food rather than when they leave his home range. (The details of the interactions of all parties are important in this case.)

6.6   TERRITORIALITY AND FLOCKING-SCHOOLING AS ALTERNATIVES

Shifts from territoriality to flocking-schooling occur both under increased predator pressure and when food competitors are territorial. These two circumstances are likely to be assessed differently. The territorial defense of food competitors could be assessed by their behavior alone. There would be no advantage to some sort of built-in response to the mere presence of the conspecific; it would be better to evaluate his behavior. The rate of attacking and threatening by the competitor would reveal its territoriality. On the other hand, waiting to learn about predators from experience could be costly, so the assessment process is more likely to include some sort of built-in response to perceiving the predator. A built-in response could take the form of being made anxious by novel stimuli. The relative rareness of predators might make such a response bias sufficient. However, a simple habituation paradigm would not do; frequent predator visits should produce a more anxious individual than infrequent visits.

Changes in response to these two different ecological circumstances may have a common mechanism. Anxiety aroused by predator presence or food competitor attacks could be reduced by the presence of conspecifics as I have already proposed in the earlier discussion of grouping as an alternative to solitary living.

6.7   ASSESSMENT PROCESSES THAT MIGHT LEAD TO ALTERNATIVE MATING SYSTEMS

The critical variable that seems to drive acorn woodpecker breeding systems is the availability of acorn storage sites, so these must somehow be assessed. The adaptive shift of males in some species from monogamy to polygyny appears to depend on each male assessing the number of territorial neighbors he has. The shift from one to several female red foxes in a particular area appears to depend on assessment of the abundance and patchiness of the resources.

Acorn woodpeckers could assess the abundance of storage sites by somehow recording the ratio of successful to unsuccessful storage attempts, or measuring the time it takes to store an acorn. Female red foxes might assess the patchiness of resources by monitoring the variation in the rates at which food is encountered during what amounts to transects across the home range. (See chapter 5 for further discussion of potential assessment mechanisms.)

The changed behavior of the female produces a shift from monogamy to polyandry, so she must assess her circumstances. California quail in many areas produce more young after a winter of high rainfall (Botsford *et al.*, 1988; Leopold, 1977; Francis, 1965). A female could assess each year's potential for adaptive polyandry via the sensory experience of the rainfall. Moreover, when rainfall is high plants grow rapidly. Rapidly growing plants have a different texture and chemical composition from normally growing plants. Both the rapid growth and the physical-chemical differences could provide the basis for assessment through sensory experience or physiological changes. In addition when more plants grow, quail eat faster and may be in better physical condition, both potential sources of assessment information.

Yet another source of assessment for female California quail is the behavior of unmated males. Adult males nearly always outnumber females. These males both approach mated pairs and vocally advertise their availability (Leopold, 1977). There is evidence that their calling increases when ecological conditions are favorable for breeding (Leopold, 1977). Females could assess ecological conditions and/or male availability by monitoring the calling rate of unmated males.

Arctic breeding shorebirds have several sources of information to draw upon. Polyandry is most common in years when the snow and ice melt early so the abundant invertebrates they feed on become available early (Schamel & Tracy, 1977). The early food availability facilitates polyandry. Day length changes markedly during the breeding season and so indexes the season's stage.

Cooperative simultaneous polyandry might be based on different assessment processes. Saddle-backed tamarin males assessing their circumstances could experience food stress and their infants' condition. The effectiveness of their intruder defense might also be a source of information to mated males assessing the adaptiveness of accepting a partner. The expression of alternative systems in naked mole rats does not seem to require an assessment mechanism.

6.8   POSSIBLE PROCESSES FOR MATING SYSTEM CHANGE

6.8.1   Monogamy and polygyny as alternatives

As noted earlier, change might be produced directly by the circumstances. But in many cases change in social systems will be a consequence of change in social predispositions.

When population density or group size increase, the interactions of breeding class males may increase. High levels of such social interactions may suppress the androgenic hormone levels of subordinate males and decrease their efforts to breed or compete for females. Different levels of effort by different sets of males would tend to facilitate breeding systems skewed toward a few males, such as polygyny and promiscuity. Northern harrier females are more attracted to males that display more, and those males are more likely to be polygynous (Simmons, 1988b). Males display more in years when voles are abundant. This mechanism might reflect (1) the better nutritional condition of the males, (2) less time devoted to foraging and more to displaying, and (3) the assessment by the males that food is available. In a somewhat similar way, sharp gradients between patches of resources in a territorial system may cause males with no access to the good patches to be relatively malnourished. Such malnourished males may tend to drop out of the breeding competition.

High predator pressure in a particular area might favor female groups. Females may assess predator pressure in several ways: seeing predators, hearing predators, or prey alarm calls. Following such an assessment they might be more anxious. If their anxiety were reduced by the presence of conspecifics they would form groups (the geometry for the selfish herd hypothesis (Hamilton, 1971) requires some such property). Female groups would favor polygyny by making them a resource males could defend.

A related change process could operate through the rate females feed or fill their stomachs or crops. If food is abundant the females could experience a high rate of stomach filling and use that experience as an assessment process. These circumstances could also support a change mechanism. Females with a lot of food available might be less likely to compete directly over a bit of food and so be more likely to tolerate one another. In species in which males would be more likely to be valued as a working parent when food was scarce, such increased female – female tolerance would make females more likely to tolerate one another in a male's territory and so become polygynous. Similarly, females foraging in rich patches would remain longer and move more slowly while foraging. This would make them more familiar with that area and so might cause females in a patchy environment to settle in proximity.

These processes could produce polygyny in altricial birds and medium sized canids by generating female clumping based on better nest sites, etc., since personal distance would have lower priority. In the real world it might well be correlated with higher predator pressure, since abundant food might lead to high concentrations of prey which could in turn increase predator presence. Thus the two factors could act together to increase the clumping of females and thus increase the likelihood of polygyny.

6.8.2 Monogamy and polyandry as alternatives

There are at least two possible change mechanisms that might account for serial polyandry as an alternative to monogamy. The first assumes that the physiological state of the female determines her response to courtship. In that case, she might recover to breeding condition more rapidly in a good year (California quail) or over a longer season (red phalarope). In breeding condition she would be responsive to courtship from a normally courting male and become facultatively polyandrous. An alternative mechanism would be that in particularly good years unattached male California quail may court more vigorously, thus stimulating a response in a physiologically identical female. Alternatively or additionally, California quail and Arctic breeding shore birds may be internally modified by a hormonal response to external stimuli or to foraging feedback.

Simultaneous polyandry in separate nests could be produced from monogamy if better nourished females are less attached to their nests and cease to relieve the male at the nest. Alternatively, better nourished males might be more reluctant to yield incubation to the female. A different mechanism probably produces simultaneous polyandry in communal nests as an alternative to monogamy. Perhaps the females are open to bonding during a certain period. If the males are already mutually tolerant, the female may enter a multiple bond with all the males that court in that short period. The prerequisite increased male–male tolerance might be produced by individual histories. Harris hawks, for example, may hunt cooperatively (Mader, 1979; Bednarz, 1988). If so, male hunting partners might have become tolerant enough to court a female simultaneously.

6.9   ASSESSMENT MECHANISMS FOR PARENTAL CARE ALTERNATIVES

6.9.1   Communal breeding and helpers at the nest

Communal breeding systems and systems of helpers at the nest are often correlated with ecological or demographic variables that favor grouping (e.g., high predation) or prevent dispersal (e.g., habitat saturation).

Alternation between one- and two-parent systems is often correlated with differences in the abundance and distribution of food.

There are a number of potential sensory sources of assessment information. Habitat saturation, for example, can be experienced in at least two ways. The social experiences of a fledged bird or grown coyote that begins to cross the boundaries of its natal territory and encounter neighbors will be a direct function of how densely conspecifics occupy the habitat. If it is well saturated they will be attacked often and everywhere. (Note that this only occurs in territories vigorously defended after the young are fledged.) In contrast, a steep gradient of resources may be experienced as a rapid decrease in certain kinds of stimulation. For example, if food or cover is a major determinant and is distributed with a steep gradient, a searching individual will find its rate of encounter suddenly decreasing or increasing.

Predators may be experienced via their sight, sound or smell. Prey that reproduced year-round or bred in a system which developed after the predation rate was established could assess the abundance of these stimuli without any special search for them. Communal care in the groove-billed ani, however, may require a different assessment process. In this case the care-giving pattern is determined before the nest is established. Therefore the assessment must take place earlier. There are two possible scenarios: in the first the communal nest is composed of pairs that have already experienced nest predation in an earlier attempt. The second is some process that assesses predator abundance by counting the predators encountered. Since nocturnal snakes are the primary nest predator, they would be most effectively counted by an animal that actively sought them out.

Many of the assessment mechanisms postulated in this chapter involve an active rather than a passive organism. This is because the needs that must be met by the social system selected are those of the young rather than those of the adult, and in some respects those needs are different. Even more than in other potential assessment mechanisms, this sort of assessment requires that the animal search for information rather than simply go about its other business and note what happens while it does so. Such an active search process is more readily handled by cognitive learning than by the S – R paradigm.

Potential helpers could assess their prospects for raising their inclusive fitness by experiencing the activity of the young and the parents. Nestlings being fed enough to optimize their survival and growth rate should beg less than deprived nestlings, and prospective helpers could also monitor their begging rate (Dow, 1979b). They could monitor the feeding rate by observing the rate parents visited the nest. A young jackal could evaluate its prospects of increasing sibling survival by monitoring the percentage of time the young are left unguarded by the parents. Similarly, young that could benefit from parasite removal could be assessed by inspection for parasites. Alternatively, the potential helper could monitor its own level of ectoparasitism and use that as an index of the young's ectoparasitism.

Parents could assess the potential net value of tolerating helpers in several ways. Like the potential helpers, they could assess the optimality of the feeding rate of the young by monitoring their behavior and appearance, and their degree of ectoparasitism by examination or by analogy to their own. The parent's own condition might also serve as an index of the cost-benefit tradeoffs of accepting help. For example, the orange-footed scrub fowl (*Megapodius reinwardt*) could assess its own fatigue or loss of condition to evaluate information about the adaptiveness of accepting another pair of parents at the same mound.

6.9.2   Two-parent and one-parent or brood split as alternatives

There are a number of experiences that could provide the information needed to assess the adaptive value of a two-parent system *vis-à-vis* one-parent or brood split systems. If one-parent care is an adjustment to food abundance the parent can experience that as the ratio of time spent hungry compared to satiated or the rate of encountering prey suitable for the young. When the parents and the young use different food, parents must actively seek information. The capability of conducting such a search for someone else's food supply could constrain adaptive modifications of such systems. The parent could also experience the young's need state via the rate at which they solicit food. One can imagine that a brood parasitic cuckoo (*Cuculus canorus*) would tend to maintain a two-parent system in foster parents that are very small and must work hard to feed the larger parasite. They could assess predation intensity by experiencing the rate of encountering the sight, sound, smell, etc., of predators and, in some cases, by the nest predation rate experienced in previous breeding attempts.

In contrast, brood split might occur as an alternative to two-parent care in response to reduced predator presence, which might act as a signal that a more efficient brood split system is a viable option.

6.10   CHANGE MECHANISMS FOR PARENTAL CARE ALTERNATIVES

6.10.1   Communal and helpers at the nest as alternatives to parental care

Intraspecific variation in social systems at the level of populations can be produced by natural selection, which would then act both as the mechanism of assessment and the mechanism of change. This mechanism will operate slowly and limits phenotypic flexibility, but it has the advantage that it avoids the costs involved in phenotypic flexibility mechanisms (see chapter 7) and it can respond to ecological variables that are difficult to assess phenotypically.

The predisposition of juveniles that remain in their parents' territory to help may be increased in various ways. Competitive motivations, such as increased aggressiveness correlated with one's own breeding effort, might be reduced. Consequently, they might be more receptive to the young as stimuli.

Despite their appearing in contradictory circumstances some of these alternative care-giving systems may have common psychological mechanisms. Increased exposure to care solicitation by young may be the mechanism in several cases. In saturated habitats juveniles may have few opportunities to disperse. Consequently they will experience solicitation by succeeding young (Dow, 1979b). Dow (1979a) put forward a model of facultative and obligate helping and communal breeding. This model uses three classes of determinants. He proposed that facultative species are more responsive to facilitation and attraction than are other species.

Many cases of facultative communal care or helpers at the nest appear in territorial species. Parents in such species have not been strongly selected to discriminate among care-soliciting young because they are unlikely to encounter young that are not their own. Therefore, in normally territorial species the threshold for response to soliciting young should be low. This would avoid rejection of own young in species that are unlikely to encounter other young. A modest amount of solicitation might stimulate parental behavior in such species. Circumstances that increase the likelihood of juveniles or adults from such species encountering young not their own are likely to produce communal care or helpers at the nest. This mechanism could operate in the same way in different ecological circumstances. Chronically hungry young might solicit non-breeding colonial birds more often in a colony than if nests were dispersed. The increased solicitation might cross a higher psychological threshold for parental care and so stimulate feeding in nonparental birds.

Increased food supply might facilitate care systems by other consequences. One is the greater risk of predation on young from a build-up of the carnivore community due to increased prey. This may increase conspecific tolerance by the same means that flocking may be produced by increased predator pressure. If increased tolerance between adults occurs in normally solitary animals not selected to discriminate among soliciting young, communal care may be a by-product of flocking. This may help to account for communal care by brown hyenas. Their case may also involve another mechanism for increased mutual tolerance that could facilitate communal care. When prey density increases, carrion feeding animals may need more carrion defense. That sometimes produces cooperative defense (Bekoff & Wells, 1980; Packer 1986). Cooperative defense might increase the mutual tolerance of adults that communal care requires (Packer, 1986).

Female mice sometimes form communal nests and suckle the young indiscriminately (Mihok, 1979), usually in cold weather. Pooling the young would pool their heat. The mothers' readiness to pool could have been selected as a response to her own body heat loss.

6.10.2 One-parent care as an alternative to two-parent care

Several possible mechanisms might produce one-parent systems as an alternative to two-parent systems when more food is available. Increased food eventually increases intraspecific competition. In territorial species this is likely to require more territorial defense, usually by the male. This takes more time, and the motivational states appropriate to territorial defense may be incompatible with parental care. The male might spend too much time actively defending and aggressively aroused to give significant paternal care. Moreover, increased food supply is often associated with a polygynous mating system. Such a system requires more male time courting and in a state of courtship arousal, both also likely to reduce paternal care. Moreover, an increased food supply is likely to make female foraging more efficient. This might reduce solicitation by the young, thus reducing the stimulation of the male's parental behavior in some species. (This assumes that males have a higher threshold than females.)

Two-parent care may be produced in overwintering male mice by the increased frequency of encounters with young. Infant rats and mice can stimulate unrelated males to provide components of parental care (Noirot, 1972).

Parents in poor physiological condition sometimes abandon their young. If one parent were in worse condition than the other, that parent's abandoning would produce the one-parent system observed in killdeer (Lenington, 1980).

The brood splitting as an alternative to two-parent care observed in grebes may be produced by a mechanism peculiar to their biology. Grebes do not fly during the breeding season. Therefore, food must be transported to the young by swimming, which is slow and has high energy costs. Grebes often have two chick broods. The chicks are carried to the foraging area on their parents' backs. When they are developed enough to float and swim, they are left on the surface while the parents dive for fish. The scarcer and less patchily distributed the fish, the more likely the parents are to make catches at a distance from one another. Since one chick is fed at a time, a parent surfacing at a considerable distance could draw the nonfeeding chick toward it, producing a situation in which the chicks were far apart but each was much nearer one parent and so was fed by that parent. A few hours of such exclusive interactions might create an exclusive relationship between each of two chicks and a particular parent. Thus, the low mobility of grebes in this phase of their lives may predispose them toward brood splitting.

6.11   STUDIES OF PROXIMATE MECHANISM OF ASSESSMENT AND CHANGE

6.11.1   Conceptual issues

The discovery and description of assessment and change processes are challenging and rewarding. There are undoubtedly many distinctive processes, but their study will usually incorporate certain general approaches and strategies.

While assessment will often (perhaps always) be revealed by changes that follow it, change itself can be studied more directly. Recall that the change we are concerned with is the change from a predisposition to interact in one way to a predisposition to interact in another way. At least some of these changes will prove to have been produced by developmental processes. Therefore, in searching for models to study these processes we should attend particularly to instances in which there are two quite different social systems and each of them develops quickly. Each of these systems should be manifested by some clearly observable events that will permit quantitative comparison of the processes producing the different relationships, and hence the different social system outcomes.

It is seldom possible to follow ideal research strategies, but it may still be useful to have ideal strategies in mind while setting out to make the best of existing opportunities and resources. In that spirit, I suggest one such strategy in three steps. The first step will be to identify an adaptive instance of intraspecific variation in social systems in which determinant(s) (e.g., ecological variables) are known. The most efficient way to take the step will probably be to peruse the literature.

The second step would be to manipulate the known determinants to produce social system change. At the same time the determinants are manipulated, several likely mechanisms (processes) should be monitored. For example, blood could be taken and hormone titers recorded.

The third and final step would be to develop hypotheses from the results of monitoring processes in stage 2, then manipulate these processes (e.g., by hormonal implants) and see if social system variation appears.

In a previous discussion of intraspecific variation in social systems (Lott, 1984) I strongly recommended more research on the proximate mechanisms involved. The studies that follow (Lott & Lott, in prep.; Lott, in prep.) were attempts to follow my own advice. They may have taught me more about the nature of such research than about the particulars of the proximate mechanisms in the systems we set out to study; in any case, it is the lessons I learned about such research that I will emphasize here.

6.11.2 Study 1: proximate analysis of territorial behavior relaxation in sunbirds

We wanted to discover the assessment process sunbirds were using. One could imagine that the process was cognitive, with the bird developing and regularly updating a mental representation of nectar levels based on the sensory experiences of foraging. An alternative is that nectar levels were not stored mentally but rather were effective via some other change in the bird's internal state. Since a direct and close correlate of the abundance of nectar in the flowers is the nectar ingested by the foraging bird, the way in which that correlate was stored and processed is a strong candidate to be a key component of the proximate assessment process. Thus, we could imagine that the level of nectar in the flowers could be assessed in at least two different ways, and we needed to think of observations that would support one or the other of those two possibilities.

A sunbird foraging in flowers with a particular nectar content has a number of experiences which the assessment process might use. These experiences range from the perception of the amount of nectar obtained in a single feeding at a single flower to changed internal states produced by ingested nectar, such as increased blood sugar level, changed insulin level, increased stomach loading, etc. A correlate of nectar levels in the flowers is the rate of ingestion of nectar and the rate of change in internal states as a consequence of nectar ingestion. Perhaps the most adaptive assessment process would respond directly to the levels of nectar in the flowers, but we know these mechanistic connections may not be perfect (e.g., oxygen and respiration rate).

In nature these correlates tend to co-occur. High levels of nectar in each flower fed from are correlated with rapid rates of ingestion, rapid rates of change in internal states such as blood sugar levels and stomach loading, and high absolute levels of such internal states. If the animals could be induced to feed from a source other than the flowers themselves, their internal state and the rate of change in their internal state would be decoupled from the level of nectar in the flowers. Since a simple sucrose solution is similar to nectar, a bird feeding from a functionally unlimited sucrose solution in an artificial feeder would have the internal state, and rate of change in internal state, of a bird feeding from superabundant nectar supplies in flowers. If this bird were also feeding from flowers that did not contain superabundant nectar supplies it would, at the same time, be getting information about the flowers. One could then compare the impact of each of these two variables on the assessment process. L. Wolf recommended we study the bronzy sunbird, which habituates well to both humans and their artifacts, and it proved an excellent choice.

In this case the assessment process is postulated because of a change in territorial behavior. We operationally defined territoriality by quantifying some of the observable features of territorial behavior. Territorial individuals should be present more of the time, they should be more likely to attack competitors that intruded into their home range, and their attacks should occur after shorter latency. We compared the rate and duration of these behavioral responses when birds were getting supplements of sugar water and when they were not.

By all these measures the birds we were observing were less territorial when they were feeding both from flowers and from a sugar-water bottle with an unlimited supply of sucrose, than when they were feeding only on such flowers (Lott & Lott, in prep.). This suggests that the assessment process is at least partially a response to internal states and or rates of change of internal states.

This study incorporates several properties that seem likely to be general features of assessment research: (1) correlates of assessment are manipulated to untangle their particular role, (2) change of social behavior was the window through which assessment was viewed, and (3) we needed an operational definition of a social system so the social systems of the manipulated and unmanipulated animals could be compared.

6.11.3   Study 2: mountain goat group size

The mountain goats of western North America (*Oreamus americanus*) live solitarily or in small groups, but larger groups are occasionally seen. These large groups are most often seen when the animals are not on near-vertical rock surfaces where they are less vulnerable to wolves (Chadwick, 1983); von Elsner-Schack, 1986).

What proximate mechanism might increase group size on less vertical surfaces? It might be that the individuals are equally inclined to be in large groups all the time, but in open habitat that preference frequently leads to larger groups for purely mechanical reasons. Alternatively, the preferred group size might shift with changes in the degree of 'riskiness' (Hennessy, 1986) experienced in different habitats. The degree of riskiness might produce an internal change in the animal that would be manifested in behavior leading to a change in the size of groups in which the animal spent its time.

One change in behavior that would produce larger groups would be an increased tendency to remain close to conspecifics. It should be adaptive for mountain goats to have evolved a psychological property that could lead to such an increased tendency to stay close in more dangerous places. Such a property could take the form of an increase in anxiety in open areas that is reduced by proximity to conspecifics. The more anxious such individuals are, the more predisposed the groups are to fusion rather than fission, so they should get larger.

Here, then, was a specific hypothesis about a proximate mechanism that produces large groups in more open habitat. To test this hypothesis I needed to observe the behavior of mountain goats in both more and less vulnerable circumstances, and see if their behavior indicated a difference in the level of anxiety in the different settings. A population of mountain goats on Mt. Evans, Colorado inhabits both steep and relatively flat areas above the timberline.

This study needed an operational definition of anxiety. Since the point of postulating anxiety was to account for animals being close together I wanted an operational definition that involved proximity. The operational definition of anxiety I chose is following distance – the distance an individual is willing to fall behind a group. The use of this measure requires the assumptions that the individual's anxiety increases directly with the distance from conspecifics, and that the individual will have a stronger tendency to reduce that distance when it is more anxious.

I located the mountain goats on slopes of different steepnesses and recorded two distances: the distance the rearmost member of a foraging group allowed to open between him and the nearest conspecific before closing it, and the distance to which he closed that gap when he did move forward. I observed that the steeper the slope the goats were on, the greater was each of these distances. Assuming that less anxious goats allowed greater distance between them and their nearest conspecific, I interpreted this as demonstrating that the steeper the slope they were on, the less anxious the mountain goats were. A second assumption was that goats further apart were more likely to experience group fission and end up in smaller groups. With these assumptions I could account for the observed difference in group size by the assumed site specific level of anxiety induced by site specific vulnerability.

6.12   SUMMARY

The study of proximate causes of intraspecific variation in social systems may involve either external events or internal mechanisms or both. From another perspective they involve either assessment or change. Change and assessment are fairly easy to distinguish in the abstract, and that distinction is useful. However, in specific cases they may be much more difficult to distinguish. The study of proximate causes may profit from careful use of postulated internal states, both physiological and psychological.

7

Intraspecific variation in social systems as an evolved strategy

Intraspecific variation in social systems is an aggregate term referring to a set of outcomes produced by a set of independent mechanisms. These outcomes are similar in conceptually important ways. I have argued that the social system alternative expressed in a particular situation usually fits that situation better than those not expressed. I have also suggested that this general mode of adjustment has been selected in the evolutionary history of the species through selection of a number of diverse mechanisms that have this general outcome in common. It is useful to consider this feature of animals as an evolved property.

This chapter addresses several questions about the evolutionary background of intraspecific variation. First I consider the application of the concept of adaptation to instances of such variation, then the costs and benefits of the sort of mechanisms that would have to operate to produce such variation. Finally, I discuss the organismic and environmental variables that make mechanisms which produce variation more or less likely to evolve in a particular species.

7.1   INTRASPECIFIC VARIATION IN SOCIAL SYSTEMS AS AN ADAPTATION

Variation in social systems is a regular feature of the biology of many species and in many cases increases fitness. This leads us to suspect that many particular instances of it are manifestations of adaptations. Simply demonstrating that a social system increases fitness does not demonstrate that it is an adaptation. As we have seen in our discussion of mechanisms, these social systems are the result of the operation of some selected process. When we can establish that the outcome of such a process is a social system that confers greater fitness, the process becomes a candidate for recognition as an adaptation.

Adaptations are central to the interest of biologists and were so well before Darwin offered the current explanation for their occurrence: natural selection (Darwin, 1859). Nevertheless, the definition and recognition of adaptation remains a thorny problem in biology. A close fit between a species' traits and its circumstances suggests the traits were designed to fit the circumstances. This criterion of design is central to the problem of recognizing adaptation (Lewontin, 1979). But, there is a tendency to equate fitness with adaptation. Many papers in the current literature describe fitness and assert adaptation. In fact, some authors have argued that fitness and adaptation are really the same thing (e.g., Clutton-Brock & Harvey, 1984).

However, I endorse the more general view (Williams, 1966; Lewontin, 1979) that evidence for design is a requirement for designation as an adaptation. In general, design in instances of intraspecific variation in social systems will be revealed by analysis of the trait that produces the variation, rather than the social systems it facilitates. This property may be either general or specific. It will usually be manifest in the mechanism by which social system variation is produced.

Territorial behavior of orange-footed scrub fowl varies via a trait that gives some evidence of design for just that variation. The orange-footed scrub fowl is an Australian mound builder with highly variable incubation techniques (Crome & Brown, 1979). 'It is known to lay eggs in beach sand, earth, fissures, between rocks and in well constructed mounds, heat for incubation coming from the sun, volcanic sources or fermentation . . .' (p. 111). Where Crome & Brown studied them nearly all the mounds were constructed in the shade and incorporated leaf litter which furnished incubation heat through fermentation. The orange-footed scrub fowl lives in a pair territory. However, in this population this social organization incorporated a surprising twist. Four of the 27 mounds were occupied simultaneously by both the pair in whose territory a shared mound was located and by a pair from a neighboring territory. The pairs did not confront each other on the mound. If one pair was working the mound when the other pair approached, the approaching pair called and the working pair left, whether they were the owners of that territory or were from the neighboring territory. Few such encounters were actually observed, since the pairs tended to work the mound on alternate days.

It is easy to construct an adaptive interpretation of this variation. Mound building and maintenance are energetically expensive. At the most studied mound, the male of one pair was working 24% of the total observation hours and the female 17%, even though the mound and its maintenance was being shared with another pair. These shared mounds occurred where there was little plant material to be incorporated into the mound. In this situation the energy to work the mound may have been a limiting resource. If so, the benefits of achieving the economies of scale that would appear likely in sharing the work of mound building could exceed the costs of the extra competition for other resources, especially since both pairs seem to have confined their feeding to their respective territories.

If this cost-benefit analysis is correct, it makes the relationship between the pairs sharing the mound seem adaptive to both, but it does not offer evidence that it is designed to do that, i.e., that it is an adaptation. However, the form of the interaction between the pairs that makes the variation possible offers some such evidence. A general rule of conduct in the relations between residents and intruders in territorially organized animals is that the residents stand fast and the intruders retreat. Indeed, that is inherent in the definition of territorial organization. A rule of conduct in which an animal present always gives way to an interloper is rare (Maynard Smith, 1976; Dawkins, 1976). Yet it is the shift from a rule in which the resident always stands fast to one in which it always yields to a particular interloper (but not to interlopers in general) that makes this alternative social system work. We seem justified in calling this shift in rules of conduct an adaptation in the rigorous sense, since evidence for design is strong.

This is a case in which the evidence for design is the presence of an attribute that is specific and appears likely to have been added to the repertoire of the birds to make intraspecific variation possible. This is a behavioral analog of Gould & Lewontin's deviation from allometric norms as evidence for adaptation (Gould & Lewontin, 1979). This is a good illustration of satisfying evidence for design, but the evidence for design in other traits which support intraspecific variation will not always be so clear-cut. For one thing, traits are likely to vary over a wide range of specificity. Recall that females androgenized in the uterus are somewhat more aggressive (vom Saal & Bronson, 1980). This increased aggression will affect many of their social interactions. The differences in interactions may be great enough to produce different relationships and different social systems in a particular set of circumstances.

A much more general mechanism would be a change in behavior via classical or operant conditioning. These are general properties involved in many of an animal's adjustments to life. The very breadth of their effect would make it difficult to demonstrate that they were designed to produce social plasticity in general, let alone any particular social system alternative. In the cases of such broadly effective mechanisms the path that evolution may have taken, and that the search for design would have to follow, would be in the relaxation of more specific social predispositions. This would allow a broadly acting trait (such as conditionability) to influence the course of the individual's development in a way that would lead to variation in social systems. It is hard to imagine how the question of design could be addressed in such a situation.

The argument to this point supposes that all responses are equally conditionable whether operantly or classically. We know that they are not. Garcia & Koelling (1966) have demonstrated a great deal of species specificity in conditioned food aversion. Rats are especially tuned to associate taste with gastric distress, but they do not establish a connection between visual stimuli and illness; quail readily associate illness with visual stimuli but do not associate illness with the taste of food (Garcia & Koelling, 1966; Bolles, 1970).

There is also species specificity in operant conditionability. Breland & Breland (1967) found dogs readily conditioned to run for food reinforcements while cows would not run for a food reinforcement but would run to avoid punishment. They note these differences are appropriate to the natural history of each species. Dogs have been selected to get food by running after it: they feed on food that has been selected to escape. In contrast, cows were selected to feed on food with little nutrition per unit of mass and that does not flee. Hence it is adaptive for cows to approach food slowly to maximize the cost-benefit ratio of obtaining and eating it.

This kind of adaptive specificity in social conditionability has not yet been demonstrated, but that may be largely because it hasn't been looked for. A search for learning processes that support social behavior might reveal a great deal of species specificity.

7.2   COSTS AND BENEFITS OF INTRASPECIFIC VARIATION IN SOCIAL SYSTEMS

I have presented a number of instances of intraspecific variation that can plausibly be interpreted as adjustments that increased the fitness of the animals that made them. After this implicit argument for the benefits of social plasticity, one might expect every species would be ready to change from any social system to any other at any time. Perhaps we Western humans, who often prefer social plasticity over rigidity in ourselves, are biased toward that view. But animals do not seem infinitely plastic, and upon reflection there are some good reasons why we should not expect them to be. It is appropriate, then, to begin our consideration of intraspecific variation in social systems as an evolved strategy with a look at its costs.

There is no *a priori* reason to suppose every instance of variation will have had its origin in some evolved, and therefore adaptive, strategy. As I have noted before, simple psychopathology will best account for some of the instances of intraspecific variation in social systems observed. Whether or not that applies in a particular instance may prove difficult to determine.

In the meantime we need to explore another source of intraspecific variation: instances in which the flexibility observed is part of an adaptive strategy in which the benefits of flexibility have outweighed the costs in evolutionary time. The following discussion assumes the flexibility we have observed is part of an overall adaptive socioecological strategy. The goal of this discussion, then, is to employ cost-benefit analysis to evaluate variation in social systems as an adaptive strategy. I approach it by comparing flexibility and inflexibility as strategies.

The comparative approach is a possible way to analyze the costs and benefits of intraspecific variation. We would compare species that do not vary in their social systems with those that do. This is similar to the usual socioecological approach to evaluating particular social systems. While this approach is logically sound, it appears to be premature. Its implementation requires that we know whether or not a particular species has the potential to vary its social system adaptively. At the present time we know that some species are able to, but we do not know if that is the case for many other species.

It would be possible to study the potential of species to express intraspecific variation in social systems. This question could be pursued intensively by studying a species in sets of circumstances systematically chosen to expose the adaptive expression of social plasticity. If the sets of circumstances needed were not encountered in nature but are probably encountered by this species in other times and places, they could be produced experimentally. Changes in the social system produced in such circumstances would be convincing, but failure to see a change would not demonstrate the species was unable to express the alternative social system. Negative results would demonstrate only that the species did not have a mechanism for the expression of intraspecific variation that worked in those particular circumstances. Thus, while it is likely that a number of species do not show flexibility, demonstrating inflexibility requires proving a negative, a difficult thing to do in something as complex as a biological system. The most we can do at this point is demonstrate that within the range of variation in social system determinants in which we have observed the animal functioning, it expressed only one system. (This issue is discussed at greater length in chapter 8.)

An alternative beginning approach to analyzing the costs and benefits of social system plasticity as an adaptive strategy is to start *de novo* and conduct an a priori (arm chair) analysis of features of intraspecific variation we can expect to operate as costs and benefits. While such analysis is certain to be incomplete, it will make us more aware that social system variation has both costs and benefits, and that both will be tied to real events, traits and processes. Moreover, we know enough about the behavior and ecology of some species to generate hypothesized costs and benefits close enough to reality to be useful.

7.3   COSTS

As I have already noted in the chapter on intraspecific variation mechanisms, an adaptive change in social systems must depend on an accurate assessment of the animal's circumstances. One of the major costs of intraspecific variation seems likely to be in the assessment process itself. However, this will depend on the mechanism operating. If the mechanism is genetic differences between populations, then the assessment process is built into natural selection, which is also the process that changes the behavior. There may be other mechanisms of social system variation in which the process of assessment is identical with the mechanism for change, but it seems likely there will be many more in which assessment and change are separate processes. In those cases, at least, assessment will impose distinct costs.

7.3.1   Costs of accurate assessment

A usefully accurate assessment requires some sort of investment in the ability to make the assessment. This investment could take several forms. One form is the devotion of a portion of the individual's general-use neurons to the storage of information useful in making decisions about the sort of social system in which to be engaged. Some part of the individual's display organs or display behavior may be devoted to the process of assessing the state of the current social system in order to determine the best social strategy to pursue.

The costs of assessment may range considerably. In most cases, more accurate assessments are likely to be more costly. Information gathered incidently to other essential activities, such as going to water once a day, may impose no additional costs. Similarly, an animal developing slowly over a long time in a stable social and ecological environment has plenty of opportunity to 'absorb' information needed for assessment, especially in a sedentary species. This would apply to most primates. But other animals live in a more dynamic ecology. Kleptoparasitic jaegers breed in the Arctic every year. When lemmings are abundant, all-purpose territories are flexible. When they are not, the birds live in coastal colonies. They must at least explore two different regions and sample foraging payoffs there. Similarly, species that are facultatively polyterritorially polygynous need to (1) leave their established territory, (2) search for a potential additional territory, (3) sample the competition for that space, and (4) determine the potential availability of additional mates, then integrate and analyze that information.

Because of these costs the potential to change adaptively will be selected only when fitness is increased by alternating social systems. However, some instances of adaptive variation may take place via properties selected for other purposes, as has the human capacity to produce calculus. Still other instances of intraspecific variation will not be adaptive, either because a process selected to produce a different social system misfired or because they were produced as artifacts of a process selected for other purposes. Even after the costs of evolving and maintaining these assessment-producing traits have been borne, employing these traits may impose still further costs. The assessment process may involve moving around in one's social and ecological environment to gather information. Movement takes time and energy and may expose the individual to risks of disease, parasitism, predation and damaging encounters with conspecifics. These costs must be borne simply to expose the animal to the stimuli that could represent information for a decision about social behavior. This information must be incorporated via something like perceptual processes and then stored in the individual for later use. This storage could be a mental representation such as memory, but it need not be. It could also be a hormonal change or a change in nutritive state that acts more or less directly on behavior. This point has been made in the discussion of mechanisms (see chapter 5).

The magnitude of the assessment cost will probably be a function of the accuracy achieved. The accuracy sought should have been selected by the tradeoffs between accuracy and cost, at least in time invested in an assessment. Even if the accuracy turns out to be a direct function of time invested, variation in the cost of being inaccurate should act back on the investment made to achieve accuracy. Therefore, some optimization process should go on. One of the things that will determine the value of accuracy is the quantitative advantage of the most optimal social system over the currently employed alternative.

These assessment tradeoffs are illustrated by a currently monogamous male bird which is evaluating the alternatives of investing parental care in his offspring and attracting another female to his territory and becoming polygynous. The relevant variables are: the number of females, his prospects of attracting one to his space, and the cost to his first brood of his shifting to polygyny instead of feeding them. The many possible variables suggest assessment could be a costly process. If each variable was assessed by a separate process that would be true. But some of the variables may have a small effect on fitness (e.g., the male's parental care may have little influence on nestling survival in this species) and so not be worth the cost of assessment. Some of the variables could be highly correlated, so assessment of the value of care would predict enough of the relevant environmental variation to make assessment of the other variables no longer cost-effective. In that case the animal should assess the variable that can be assessed at lowest cost. Reality may be harsher: in many cases when fitness from one variable increases, fitness from others will decrease (e.g., more females means fertilizing more eggs, but if nestlings cannot grow optimally without paternal care, more hatchlings means smaller fledglings).

7.3.2   Costs of erroneous assessment

The costs I have discussed so far must be borne even if the assessment is accurate, but assessment will be wrong at least part of the time. One reason faulty assessments are inevitable is that the assessment process fails to incorporate all the information necessary to make a faultless assessment. Suppose an assessment of whether or not to be territorial depended not only on the overall density of the population but also on the demographics of the population. For example, juveniles might generate much less intruder pressure than adults. However, the assessment process in use might treat all conspecifics equally. Such an assessment process would be useful in that there would be a correlation between total population and total intruder pressure, but its accuracy would vary from situation to situation as the demographics of the population varied. The degree of inaccuracy would depend on the reproductive characteristics of the species involved (e.g., r- vs. k-selected species) and the variability of the local carrying capacity.

Another source of error in the assessment process is, in a sense, purely statistical. Most, perhaps all, assessment processes depend on sampling. Unless the sample is total and is made at the instant in which the alternative social system will be implemented, it will be unrepresentative to some degree. Even if the mechanism by which the shift is made is one that can operate at the present moment, the sample used in assessment has a certain statistical probability of being wrong: the probability that the sample is by chance wrong to a particular degree. Sample size, i.e., effort in assessment, will strongly influence the magnitude of that probability.

But this is not the only potential source of error. The mechanism by which intraspecific variation in social systems occurs may have operated before the present circumstances were established. Such a mechanism will be subject to two sampling errors. The first is the sampling of the animal's circumstances at the time the mechanism operates. The second is the error inherent in needing to treat the circumstances in which the mechanism fixes the social system as a sample of the circumstances in which the social system will operate. The sampling that takes place when the mechanism operates is essentially a prospective sample of the circumstances the animal will face when the system selected is in operation. The accuracy of that forecast will influence the value of the shift, and its potential inaccuracy will be one of the costs of intraspecific variation in social systems as a strategy.

7.3.3 Costs of social system change

Even if a very accurate assessment has occurred and the costs of having assessment-making traits and using them will be repaid, there are still the costs of making the change in social interactions which produce the alternative social system. One such cost is inherent in the mechanism that will produce the change. Suppose the mechanism for change in social interactions produces it through a gradual shift in the probability of interacting in particular ways. Such a mechanism would produce fluctuating behavior that may impose high costs during transition because of its inconsistency. It is at least possible the animal will go through a stage in which it is bearing all or most of the costs of both social systems while getting none or few of the benefits of either. An example might be an animal in the process of a gradual shift from territorial to dominance organization.

If its behavior fluctuates between the two patterns, it may spend some time and energy excluding conspecifics from its territory without excluding enough conspecifics enough of the time to keep the level of foraging competition below that of an animal expressing dominance. At the same time, it could be expressing a level of dominance-producing behavior but doing so too inconsistently to maintain stable dominance relationships. It might assert itself in dominance fashion part of the time outside its former territory, then shift to a territory producing pattern and retreat from the same individual at a different time but in the same place. Such inconsistent behavior might produce little of the advantages of a dominance system; while still imposing much of the costs of a dominance system. Of course there may be situations in which an intermediate or mixed strategy is the most effective, and the animal will settle there. But, intermediate states might be a little more costly because they confuse social partners. Mixed signals may raise the cost of interacting.

A related cost is, being out of synchrony with the rest of the population. If the optimal strategy is dominance but the population is behaving territorially, the first animal to shift to a dominance-producing pattern of behavior might pay high costs, but experience low increases in fitness. While it is responding to individuals on the basis of their past history of interactions regardless of where they occurred, those individuals will be responding to it on the basis of the location of the current interaction. Each will be behaving inconsistently from the point of view of the other, but most of the cost of the confusion would be borne by the animal behaving differently. This observation is closely related to the demonstrations of Evolutionarily Stable Strategy theory that the optimal strategy depends in part on the strategies being employed by the rest of the population.

On the other hand, certain strategies can be invaded by others even when they predominate (Maynard Smith, 1976). In that case, there could be major advantages in behaving differently from the rest of the population. A possible example is when territorial behavior is no longer worthwhile and a more profitable pattern would be to shift to an undefended home range. The outcome could depend on demographics. Suppose all the members of the population had a territory. The advantage could be that the non-territorial individuals' neighbors would stay home, and he would get the benefit of the space without bearing the costs of defending it. Thus the optimal strategy would be made even more beneficial because the others in the population were pursuing a different strategy. But this would depend on circumstances: if the population were above carrying capacity, there would be many potential intruders. In that case the first animal to abandon territoriality would lose resources very rapidly to intruders still being rebuffed by other territory holders.

7.4   BENEFITS

The general way in which social plasticity can benefit an animal is by allowing it to change from a less optimal social system to a more optimal one. Sunbirds that relax their territorial behavior when nectar is superabundant forage more efficiently than if they did not. Female phalaropes that have two broods fledged in a given year, by becoming polyandrous, have higher fitness than those that have fledged only one brood. As we have seen, the costs of having and implementing the potential to express alternative social systems may be considerable, and the benefits must fully offset those and leave some net advantage for social plasticity to be favored. But even a small net edge would support favorable selection of traits creating the potential for intraspecific variation in social systems.

Earlier (chapter 2, p. 37) I contrasted the success of colonial versus solitary nesting in both black-headed and brown-hooded gulls. Mobbing is effective against carrion crows (which are solitary predators on black-headed gulls) and give colonial birds higher fitness (Patterson, 1965). Mobbing is not effective against caracaras (which hunt in cooperating pairs) so that solitary brown-hooded gulls had higher fitness (Burger, 1974).

These interactions create a situation in which social pioneers could enjoy high fitness. Take the black-headed gull colony with its carrion crow predators (Patterson, 1965) as the beginning point. Presently the great bulk of the prey biomass is unavailable to the carrion crows because they hunt alone. A change to the caracara technique by only one pair of carrion crows could transform the gull colony from a virtual desert to a superabundant source of easily obtained food. These pioneering crows would have an enormous advantage over their conspecific competitors that hunted alone, and in part that advantage would be due to the rarity of their social system. (Adopting the caracara strategy is probably essential. Montevecchi (1979) has shown that two ravens foraging in a kittiwake (*Risa tridactyla*) colony have *lower* success per individual when flying together than one.)

Now suppose some variation-producing mechanism operated with the result that this form of pair hunting over colonies became universal in carrion crows. Complete concentration of the carrion crows on the colony nests would create an opportunity for social pioneers among the black-headed gulls. They could begin to behave like some of the brown-hooded gulls in Argentina and begin to nest alone. In view of the easy plunder in the colonies the crows might concentrate their efforts there, reducing predation on the solitary gull nests to zero and giving the pioneering gulls high fitness. As more and more gulls pursued that strategy, coloniality would be abandoned and all gulls would nest solitarily.

This would create an opportunity for a pioneering change in social system by carrion crows. With more biomass now available in vulnerable, isolated gull nests, a shift to searching for those nests would be advantageous. This too could be done by the cooperating pairs, but since the solitary nests are easily taken by one crow, and since working in pairs involves the costs of sharing captured prey, it would be advantageous to hunt alone. Again, the pioneers would have an advantage. The increased fitness conferred by this pattern could lead to its being imitated by the rest of the crow population. If crows again hunted alone, gulls that pioneered a shift in social system to colonial nesting would have a decided advantage.

The point of this oversimplified scenario is to demonstrate that there are circumstances in which a different social system is advantageous just because it is different. Thus, one of the potential benefits offsetting the costs of having flexibility and implementing it is the benefit of having a different social system than one's contemporaries.

7.5   PREDICTING SOCIAL SYSTEM PLASTICITY AS A TRAIT

The foregoing discussion indicates intraspecific social system variation can be an adaptive trait when the benefits exceed the costs. The points made in that discussion should help us predict what sort of species is likely to express such variation. The predictive factors fall into two general categories, organismic variables and environmental variables. These two factors will be correlated to a degree, because environments will have selected some of the properties of animals that live in them. However, some important organismic variables will be relatively independent of environmental variables. For example, the East African savannah is one environment yet the body sizes of the largest antelopes occupying it are several times larger than the body size of the smallest antelope there (Jarman, 1974).

Body size is an organismic variable that might influence the potential to express territoriality. The costs of territorial behavior include the energy expended moving one's body about the territory to remove intruders. For large animals living on moderate quality food, e.g., large ruminants, the benefits of maintaining foraging territories will seldom outweigh the costs (Jarman, 1974). In such cases the costs of maintaining the potential to express territoriality would seldom be repaid, and that potential is not likely to have been favored by selection.

7.5.1   Ecological niche

Large niches, on the other hand, are likely to increase the value of social system variability and the probability that selection will have favored it. An omnivore capable of shifting from one kind of food to another is likely also to be shifting to foods with different distributions and renewal characteristics. A fox foraging on meadow mice would have a stably distributed resource that might well repay territorial behavior. However, a fox foraging on fruit might find each fruit source ephemeral yet superabundant when available. In that case scramble competition and undefended home ranges might be a more cost-effective strategy. This argument can also be stood on its head, however; under the circumstances, an omnivore might be able to create a stable food supply in one space by shifting its diet to seasonally available food.

The North American large-mammal fauna is depauperate compared to Africa's, while its range of habitats is similar. Consequently the 12 North American ungulates (Gilbert, 1978) might have less narrowly defined niches than the 90 African ungulates (Leuthold, 1977). If social systems contribute to niche fitting one would expect the North American ungulates to be more variable in their social systems. Pronghorn antelope,. moose (*Alces alces*), mule deer and mountain sheep are known to breed in alternative systems, as do some African antelopes. Not enough information is currently available to test this prediction, but perhaps it provides some insight into the apparently maladaptive territorial efforts of migrating wildebeest (*Connochaetes taurinus*) bulls.

An organismic variable likely to influence the way in which social system variation is expressed is the overall reproductive strategy of the species. While it is clear there are real limitations in describing species as r- or k-selected, there remains some value in recognizing that there are high and low intrinsic rates of reproduction, and that those different rates tend to be associated with other organismic variables. The mechanisms for social system variation in r-selected species seem more likely to be natural selection, while the mechanism in k-selected species seems more likely to be one that operates during the individual's life.

7.5.2   Plasticity potential

Other organismic variables may preadapt species to social flexibility. All canids can regurgitate. Canids may have evolved this trait for the immediate benefit of the individual, e.g., as a way to eliminate toxic meat. But since partially digested meat is a good food source for young canids, this property allows males to feed their young more directly than most other male mammals. This, in turn, creates additional potential for cost-effective male care, and may help account for much of the mating-system plasticity common in canids (Moehlman, pers. comm.).

One might expect the impressive intellectual talents of primates to support a great deal of social plasticity. Yet intraspecific variation in social systems is not frequently reported in primates (Wrangham, 1983). Perhaps high intellectual function is not a common mechanism for social system plasticity and may not be a particularly useful one. Alternatively, it may be that primates are capable of a great deal of intraspecific variation but are usually seen in stable circumstances where social system variation is not stimulated.

7.5.3   Environmental stability

If the environment changes rapidly and frequently, variable social systems might be favored. Certain latitudes (e.g., the North American Great Plains) have inherently unstable climates due to north-south variation in jet-stream flow (Bryson, 1974, 1980; Bryson & Murray, 1977). These climatic shifts might favor social system flexibility in animals living largely in those habitats.

Whether or not the environment is stable is partly a function of the time scale involved. The longer an animal lives the more environmental change it is likely to encounter. But it is not clear that we should expect longevity per se to favor intraspecific variation in social systems. While adult phenotypic flexibility would seem to be advantageous in an animal more likely to experience variation in the course of living a long life, a long-lived animal can tolerate a period of suboptimal functioning at less cost to lifetime reproductive success.

The rate at which forage renews as it relates to the animal's body size and required frequency of reinitiating foraging might influence the value of social system variation. So far sunbirds have shown intraspecific variation while their much smaller ecological equivalents – hummingbirds – are only rarely reported to give up territoriality. Perhaps hummingbirds cannot take the same risks of delayed feeding.

7.5.4   Versatility of present social system

The versatility of an observed social system should affect whether or not a particular species is likely to manifest social system variation. A useful definition of a versatile social system might be one in which cost-benefit ratios do not change rapidly with changes in circumstances. This definition implies that social systems are not all equally versatile, an assumption that intuitively seems correct. Dominance organization appears to be manageable in more circumstances than a territorial system, though it also seems less optimal in some of those circumstances. Similarly, the overlapping, undefended home ranges of many solitary carnivores can undergo great quantitative variation with little if any qualitative change, as home range sizes and degree of overlap vary from circumstance to circumstance (Kruuk, 1975).

7.5.5   Compatibility with other features of social and reproductive systems

Certain features of social systems facilitate shifts to alternative social systems. For example, monogamous birds in which both partners share incubation can shift to either polygyny or polyandry by making only a quantitative, not a qualitative, change in their incubation pattern. In a different way, facultative helping at the nest or den is favored by a parental mating system of long term monogamy. That breeding system increases the relatedness of the helpers to the helpees. A parental care system in which male care is not always essential facilitates the development of polygyny. In the same way, a parental care system in which female participation is not always needed permits the development of polyandry.

Similarly, features of the reproductive biology of the animals may facilitate alternative systems. The Coolidge effect (recovery of sexual motivation by previously sexually exhausted males when presented with a new partner) has been reported in a number of mammalian species (Symons, 1979). To date there are no comparable demonstrations of a similar effect in females. The Coolidge effect tends to bias males toward polygyny. Consequently its presence in a particular species would facilitate a change from monogamy to polygyny and inhibit a change from polygyny to monogamy. Of course, the Coolidge effect is likely to have been selected in a species that will benefit from polygyny.

The difference in the degree to which the reproductive success of one sex is influenced by the behavior of the other sex is another factor that may influence the potential plasticity of social systems. Martin & Hannon (1987) have observed that female ptarmigan are equally successful in monogamous or polygynous systems. Such females are not likely to employ any strategies to preserve monogamy. This would permit the development of polygyny in the males. Similarly, the frequency of facultative polyandry in shorebird mating systems is probably facilitated by the fact that females make a negligible contribution to the rearing of the young. Symons (1979) argued that women are more accepting of the variety of human mating systems than men, because variation in mating systems does not affect their reproductive success as much as it does that of males.

Intraspecific nest parasitism is a feature of many avian breeding systems and one likely to act as a constraint on parental care systems. Cooperative polygyny requires each female to accept the presence and eggs of another female in the nest. In species subject to intraspecific nest parasitism, selection would have favored females that excluded others from their nest (Andersson, 1984). Such female behavior would act as a barrier to simultaneous polygyny. Behavior that may overcome such a barrier appears to figure in one of the few known instances of facultative simultaneous, cooperative polygyny in birds. Female Galapagos mockingbirds (*Nesomimus formicivora*) joining a nest 'established their credentials' by acting as helpers with the first brood of the breeding season. They contributed eggs to the following clutches (Curry, 1988).

It may be easier for a solitary animal to shift from an undefended home range system to a territorial system than to shift to a dominance system. Many dominance systems seem to require not only working out dominance relationships but also recalling each of them. Unless animals have been selected for recalling the many relationships, they may be unable to do so. This difficulty could be even greater if the communicatory repertoire of the territory holders emphasizes information about location more than information about identity.

7.5.6   Compatibility with other features of natural history

Some features of natural history are incompatible with certain social systems. For example, the limited ability of most male mammals to increase the reproductive output of females makes polygyny a much more likely alternative to monogamy than polyandry. Circumstances that produce intraspecific variation in social systems in some species are irrelevant in others. For example, in many species flocking or schooling may be an adaptive response to the presence of a predator, but top carnivores, by definition, are never subject to that pressure.

7.5.7 Psychological complexity of shift

If individuals are to live in alternate social systems they must shift from one of them to the other. Intuitively, the more psychologically complex a shift is, the less likely it is to occur. An adaptive shift in birds from monogamy to polygyny with each female nesting separately requires only one psychological difference: male courtship of more than one female. Just as an increase in food resources can make care by both parents in a monogamous pair unnecessary and so justify polygyny, decreased resources can make the efforts of both parents inadequate and so justify cooperative polyandry as a more fit alternative than complete breeding failure. For example, the breeding success of Peruvian seabirds is profoundly and regularly affected by the Pacific Ocean upwelling failures known as El Ninos. Ordinary El Ninos reduce nesting success by more than a third, and most birds do not even attempt to breed during severe El Ninos (Duffy, 1980). The reduction in food availability clearly produces a situation in which cooperative polyandry would produce breeding success for birds which would fail monogamously, yet birds either breed monogamously or not at all.

One of the reasons for this may be that a shift to cooperative polyandry is psychologically more complex than a shift to polygyny. It requires (1) females accepting courtship from more than one male and (2) male tolerance of other males being on the same nest and copulating with the same female. This constitutes a more complex and therefore less likely shift. It has also been reported much less frequently than a shift to polygyny. Table 3.1 records 111 species reported to be polygynous as an alternative to being monogamous, while table 3.7 records only 16 species reported to be cooperatively polyandrous as an alternative to being monogamous. Both tables fall far short of a complete reporting of either variation, but each is a sufficiently unbiased sample of the current literature to permit valid comparisons of rates of occurrence.

Similarly, reports of simultaneous polygyny at a single nest in birds are much more rare than those of simultaneous polygyny at different nests in birds or in mammals. The possibility of nest parasitism mentioned above may be one reason for this, but it is also possible that the increased psychological complexity of the shift is another. Simultaneous polygyny at different nests differs from monogamy in that each female must tolerate at least one other in the same home range. Simultaneous polygyny at the same nest requires not only that tolerance in the home range, but also tolerance at the nest, and even some means of sharing incubation duties. These several differences seem to require a more complex process to reach the more different alternative.

7.5.8   Environmental constraints

The physical environment in which the animals are living may influence the readiness to express particular social systems. The degree to which the habitat is physically open or closed may act as a constraint on the type of social system implemented. The cost of keeping a large social group functioning coherently may be greater in closed habitat (e.g., forest) compared to open habitat (e.g., grassland). The locations of animals relative to one another is much more easily ascertained in an open habitat (Barrette, 1988). Perhaps this is one reason why white-tailed deer live in large groups in open habitat compared to closed habitat (Hirth, 1977) and reedbuck formed groups when their habitat was opened by a fire (Jungius, 1971). Open habitat may also facilitate the development of lekking that depends on visual advertisement, such as that of topi antelope and Uganda kob. Conversely, when the landmarks of a traditional lek are obscured by snow, sage grouse (*Centrocercus urophasianus*) breed without lekking (Gibson & Bradbury, 1987).

Other conditions that may influence the ability to advertise one's presence may also affect the ability to express particular alternative social systems. For example, European otters (*Lutra lutra*) defend territories when they occupy streams but do not defend them when they forage in the ocean. One of their principal territorial behavior patterns is scent-marking. The shorelines of streams offer many more opportunities to scent mark than do oceans. Scent marking species may also be less successful in maintaining a territory in an area washed by heavy rainfall. Also, the noise of rainfall obscures sounds, so marking territories or advertising leks with sounds may be more difficult. Naturally noisy environments are sometimes created by large aggregations of sound producing animals such as birds or insects. Some human modified environments are also noisy.

7.5.9   Demographic constraints

Demographic phenomena may determine the likelihood of intraspecific variation in social systems. Female mortality in California quail exceeds that of males (Leopold, 1977). The resulting imbalanced sex ratio facilitates the occurrence of facultative serial polyandry during years when foraging conditions make that possible. At the same time, that biased sex ratio also makes facultative polygyny unlikely.

8

Using intraspecific variation in social systems to test socioecological hypotheses

Interpretations of social behavior as an adaptation to a species' ecological circumstances have increased rapidly since the early 1960s (Eisenberg 1962, 1966; Crook, 1965) and are now widespread. Many persuasive socioecological analyses have been, and continue to be, made on large and small scales. Yet other predictions were not fulfilled (Clutton-Brock & Harvey, 1977). There can be many reasons for the failure of any hypothesis to survive a test, but in the case of socioecological hypotheses there is a persistent doubt that we have an adequate way to test them. There is a longstanding need, then, for a clear-cut way to test socioecological hypotheses. Recently, many socioecologists have turned to intraspecific variation in social systems as the long sought solution to that problem.

Such variation offers new opportunities to test socioecological hypotheses, but those opportunities are neither as numerous nor as straightforward as is often assumed. To see clearly what the problem is, and why intraspecific variation is seen as a solution, we must recall the history of socioecology. With an understanding of the problem and the reasons intraspecific variation is seen as a solution, we can go on to consider the potential of such variation to solve these problems, and the ways in which it must be used to provide a sound solution.

Socioecological theory first emerged as a series of *post hoc* explanations for a substantial body of already known data. Crook (1965) interpreted the tendency of different species of weaver birds to nest colonially or solitarily as a function of the distribution of their resources. Similarly Crook & Gartlan (1966) interpreted the grouping patterns reported to be characteristic of primate species as a function of the distribution of resources and the pattern of the predation pressures those species faced. Crook (1970) proposed a general ecological interpretation of primate social systems. Earlier Eisenberg (1966) wrote a wide-ranging review of the socioecology of mammals. In these *post hoc* interpretations, the already known social behavior of each species was analyzed as a response to the already known ecology of that species. The fit of known circumstances to known social systems was compelling, and by the late 1960s socioecology was in full stride. These *post hoc* interpretations were so plausible that the general framework they exemplified was quickly incorporated into the general world view of people working in the field.

Yet from a formal point of view, the particular relationships between ecological variables and social behavior were simply post dictions. These post dictions were a source of hypotheses ready to generate predictions that could be used to test the hypotheses. However, as these *post hoc* explanations were formalized to predictions and tested by the observation of previously unobserved species or species whose social behavior had not yet been interpreted in this framework, their predictive power was sometimes surprisingly weak. The behavior of many species simply did not fit the predictions socioecological theory seemed to make (e.g., Clutton-Brock & Harvey, 1977). In fact, it seemed at times that the power of the perspective was inversely related to the information available.

There are many reasons why a socioecological prediction might not be confirmed. Perhaps the particular prediction was an inappropriate inference from a sound socioecological hypotheses. Perhaps the deduction from theory was correct but the test of the hypotheses was not appropriate. Alternatively, the deduction and the test of the hypotheses might be correct but the behavior is not optimal. The socioecology of interspecific differences is limited to observing the results of selection and, as best as can be done, reconstructing the selection history of the observed phenomena. Attempts at rigorous testing of socioecological hypotheses, like other adaptive hypotheses, are frequently frustrated because of a reasonable and ready alternative interpretation of data that don't fit.

8.1   PHYLOGENETIC INERTIA

Phylogenetic intertia is that reasonable and ready alternative. When we evaluate tests of evolutionary predictions, we must recognize that the species has not only selection pressures at the present, but also a history of selection pressures that shaped its behavior in the past. Some of its present traits may have been selected as adaptations under other circumstances and survived into the present simply because selection has not had time or available genetic variability to change them (Clutton-Brock & Harvey, 1977; Eisenberg, 1981; Berger, 1988; Kavanau, 1988). The social behavior of domestic dogs and cats provides a good example of the explanatory use of phylogenetic inertial. The ecological circumstances of dogs and cats in human households are similar, yet the social behavior of the two species is different. We account for that difference, in good part, by invoking the differences in the niches occupied by their wild ancestors.

Yet phylogenetic inertia has a peculiar role in the understanding of social phenomena. It is usually the explanatory alternative of last resort – the explanation we offer when a persuasive predictor of an ecological variable or a social system fails. Consequently, it has little appeal to scientists. It seems to block rather than facilitate discovery, because the answer it proposes cannot be tested. But questions should not be abandoned simply because they are not immediately testable. The chemical composition of the sun once appeared to be beyond the reach of science. But once it was discovered that the chemical composition of material is revealed by the spectrum of light it emits when heated, the chemical composition of the sun was known in a few years. Moreover, while invoking phylogenetic inertia seems in some ways the last refuge of rascals, it is also perfectly legitimate.

Le Boeuf (1986) provided an example of the use of phylogenetic inertia in the interpretation of socioecological data. He reviewed the literature on mating patterns in seals and walruses and found the mating system correlates with two kinds of breeding substrate. Species breeding on islands are polygynous while species breeding on pack ice are monogamous. This makes sense because an island will remain intact through the breeding season, while pack ice will break up and the area where a group of females is gathered will fragment. Also, islands have restricted areas for breeding; this forces females to aggregate. Pack ice is virtually unlimited, allowing females to disperse. Aggregated females are more easily defended so islands facilitate polygyny.

The behavior of walruses is contrary to the predictions of this sensible analysis: they breed on pack ice but are polygynous. Le Boeuf suggested part of the solution to this puzzle may be that the ancestors of walruses lived in temperate waters where they probably bred on islands and were polygynous. The mating behavior of walruses is still influenced by this phylogenetic history, i.e., by inertia. In other words, the selection process has not had time to convert to a pattern more adaptive on pack ice. (This is only one reason Le Boeuf offered for the deviation of walruses from the trend.)

This case illustrates both the reasons for invoking phylogenetic inertia and the dissatisfaction that persists after having invoked it. The case occurs because a powerful perspective on behavior has run aground – an exception must be explained. Moreover, the use is legitimate: the ancestors of walruses probably did behave the way present walruses do. A simple failure to adjust to changed circumstances accounts for the failure of socioecological theory to predict the current species behavior.

Yet it is an explanation that gives little satisfaction. For one thing, it is invoked to explain exceptions rather than rules, things that should happen but don't. For another, the validity of the explanation is hard to determine. The very form of the hypotheses makes it hard to evaluate, beyond a determination of its basic legitimacy. Finally, it is an appeal to random rather than orderly processes. Even so, given what we know about natural selection, we can be sure that sometimes it is the appropriate explanation.

8.2 COMPARATIVE APPROACHES DESIGNED TO AVOID PHYLOGENETIC INERTIA

Thus phylogenetic inertia has become at once the salvation of particular socioecological hypotheses and the *bête noir* of socioecological theory in general. The more readily it is accepted as an explanation, the less subject to rigorous testing are the generalizations it saves. Consequently there is a need, and there has been an active search, for tests of socioecological hypotheses in which phylogenetic inertia is not such a ready and reasonably alternative interpretation of observations that do not confirm predictions. Solutions to this problem have taken two forms. Each form avoids the problem of phylogenetic inertia at the species level by making the comparisons at a different taxonomic level. One approach has been to make comparisons at a higher taxonomic level where the idiosyncracies of the history of a particular species would contribute less random variation. Clutton-Brock & Harvey (1977) reduced the random variation that phylogenetic inertia introduces into the system by making predictions about the social system of primates at the level of genera rather than species.

The second approach is to go to a lower taxonomic level and test predictions by observing differences in social systems within a species rather than between species. In other words, intraspecific variation in social systems seem to offer a solution to the phylogenetic inertia problem, and it is currently being welcomed as a means of testing socioecological theory (e.g., Rubenstein, 1986; Wrangham, 1986; Gosling, 1986). Apparently adaptive intraspecific variation often seems to confirm the predictions of socioecological theory. The close fit of golden-winged sunbirds' social systems to the economics of foraging at any one point in time confirms a long-standing prediction about the function and evolution of territoriality: a territory is defended when it is economically defensible (Brown, 1964).

With the rapid increase in recorded instances of intraspecific variation, and the general consensus that it is usually adaptive, socioecologists have turned to it more and more as a means of testing socioecological theory. I have already cited the work on sunbirds by Gill & Wolf. In a recent volume (Rubenstein & Wrangham, 1986) this approach was used implicitly by several authors. Rubenstein (1986) observed both territoriality and undefended home ranges in a single small population of feral horses. He interpreted these different patterns as adaptive responses to differences in the microecology of the island on which they were living. The males defended territories where the open habitat made intruders readily detectable, and the narrowness of the island meant the sea formed easily defended boundaries on the two long sides of the territory. He used this post diction as a general test of theoretical predictions about the distribution of resources and the expression of territoriality.

Other authors have predicted a particular form of intraspecific variation and used those predictions to make socioecology a predictive science. Wrangham (1986) proposed that the group size and degree of sociality of females is determined by the abundance of terrestrial herbaceous vegetation. He noted that currently known chimpanzee (*Pan troglodytes*) populations had little of that resource while currently known bonobo (*Pan paniscus*) groups had more of it, and the bonobos were more gregarious and lived in larger groups. He proposed to test this hypotheses by observing other populations of chimpanzees with different abundances of terrestrial herbaceous vegetation.

Gosling (1986) developed a theory of mating strategies in African antelopes. One of the predictions he made was that following would be a favored male strategy when females form social groups. He suggested this prediction could be tested by intraspecific comparisons of following behavior in populations which vary in group size.

This approach was taken to the level of an experimental test by Berger (1988). He started with the fact that Grevy's zebras (*Hippotigris grevyi*) are rarely in harems while mountain zebras (*H. quagga*) nearly always are. Grevy habitat is typically more xeric where the costs of harem defense would be relatively greater. He tested this hypothesis by manipulating the distribution of food for groups of both species in the same habitat. While both species changed their home range usage in response to food distribution changes, neither changed their social grouping patterns. Berger recognized the limitations of incomplete experiments, but cautiously (and reasonably) concluded that the persisting differences were due to phylogenetic inertia.

8.3 ASSUMPTIONS MADE WHEN TESTING SOCIOECOLOGICAL HYPOTHESES VIA SOCIAL SYSTEM VARIATION

The logic of using intraspecific variation to test socioecological hypotheses is illustrated in each of the above examples. In all cases the logic is persuasive, provided that some necessary assumptions are true. Two specific assumptions and another class of assumptions are involved. The first specific assumption is that existing social systems always optimize fitness. The second specific assumption is that the relevant ecological variables have been identified and appropriately measured. The class of assumptions relate to the subjects observed and the processes by which their social systems are determined. In the pages that follow I develop the impact of these assumptions.

8.3.1 Optimality assumptions

The first specific assumption is that the behavior observed is optimal. Socioecological theorizing sometimes consists of logically constructing the behavior pattern that would be optimal in particular ecological circumstances and predicting that it will be found there (Krebs & Davies, 1987). The investigator then looks at the animal in those circumstances to see if the prediction is borne out. When this paradigm is applied to instances of intraspecific variation in social systems an assumption is made, though not always explicitly, that when two different social systems are observed in the same species, each system confers the greatest fitness that could be observed in those circumstances; in other words, that the behavior observed is optimal.

But such observations can really only test whether or not the predictions are correct. They do not test the fitness of either the behavior predicted or the behavior observed. In fact it will be difficult to know whether or not a social system is optimal. The prediction that it is cannot be tested if a species always expresses a particular social system in a particular set of circumstances (circumstances A), because fitness must be expressed as relative to another phenotype. The true fitness of the alternative social system (the one expressed in different circumstances – circumstances B) can only be observed if expressed in A. If the predictions fail we are justified in rejecting the hypotheses only if we assume the behavior was optimal, yet we have no direct information about that. An unambiguous test of socioecological hypotheses by an instance of social system variation requires an evaluation of the relative fitness conferred by each of the alternatives in each of the sets of circumstances.

In practice, fitness itself is seldom determined in studies of social systems. Instead, some index of fitness is measured. If the index of fitness chosen can be measured directly, the evaluation of its optimality can be simple. Gill & Wolf (1975) predicted the optimal management of time and energy by golden winged sunbirds. They were able to measure and compare the time and energy costs and benefits of each of two alternative social systems in achieving that optimal management in different circumstances. According to Pyke's (1979) analysis of their data, the sunbirds managed their energy budget in a way that maximized the time spent sitting.

The comparison of social systems using other measures of fitness can be much more difficult. Consider the case in which the comparison is between two different mating systems, and the measure of fitness is the number of offspring produced. This measure in inherently relative rather than absolute. The fitness of each system is defined by its relationship to the fitness of the alternatives. The needed comparison may be difficult to achieve. If the particular alternatives always appear in particular circumstances then their fitness cannot be compared. If they do not, it will always be possible that there is some critical difference in the two sets of circumstances.

8.3.2   Ecological determinants identified assumption

A second assumption is that the only significant difference in the two observational situations being compared is the ecological variable identified as the determinant. Consider the application of this assumption in Gill & Wolf's work on golden-winged sunbirds. Here two variables were measured: the behavior of the birds and the level of nectar in the flowers from which they were feeding. Many other features of the observational situation were constant. The geographic setting was the East African Rift Valley within one degree of the equator. Sunrise and sunset were at essentially the same time every day. Temperature varied within narrow limits as a function of the progress of the seasons from dry to rainy, but even in the rainy season the daily weather regime was stable, with rain coming at a predictable time of day. The birds fed on the same species of plant (*Leonotis nepetifolia*) throughout the day and from day to day throughout the study. The density of flowers and the level of nectar in each flower varied during the study, and this variation correlated with the shift in social systems. The work by Gill & Wolf also illustrates the second aspect of this assumption – that the relevant ecological variables have been identified.

These assumptions are conceptually simple and may be made in either a strong form or a weak form. The strong form of assumption is that everything variable either has been measured or it is not a social system determinant. It is usually not expressed this way but may be inferred from the analysis and discussion of the data. The weak form of the assumption is that not all the relevant ecological variables are measured, but at least some variance in behavior is determined by the recorded variance in an ecological feature(s). For example, the only ecological factors Gill & Wolf measured were the number of flowers, the rate of nectar production, and the volume of nectar in the flowers. Intruder pressure and predation were not measured. The unstated assumption was that a meaningful amount of the variance in the expression of territoriality could be accounted for in the absence of measures of these ecological variables. In fact, nearly all the variance in behavior seemed to be explained by the few ecological variables that were measured.

8.4   EVALUATING THESE ASSUMPTIONS

There is no simple or straightforward formula for evaluating assumptions about the ecology. To do so, we must use our wits and the state of our knowledge. In one sense, the ideal approach would be to measure every variable known or suspected to produce variation in the measure under study. However, that list is likely to be long, and some of the measures are likely to be difficult. For example, I have argued that parasites and diseases might operate as ecological determinants of intraspecific social system variation. In some cases those variables might be difficult to measure. This difficulty is encountered in any field situation: there are a lot of loose variables and some may prove to be loose cannons. One approach offered by Brown *et al.* (1978) is to emphasize the use of multiple correlation techniques to evaluate the relationship between variation in social behavior and variation in ecological variables. This approach offers a level of rigor otherwise unavailable to field workers, but we must recognize that it does not address the question of the generality of the findings. Generalizing relationships demonstrated by this analysis depends on other approaches.

8.5   ASSUMPTIONS ABOUT PHYLOGENETIC INERTIA AND POPULATION DIFFERENCES

The class of assumptions about the subjects are both less familiar and more difficult to deal with. Recall that the special opportunity intraspecific variation seems to offer is that it avoids sources of uncontrollable variance that are inherent in making interspecific comparisons. The most important of these sources of variance is phylogenetic inertia. I have noted earlier in this chapter that this is an important issue in interspecific comparative analysis, and that many discussions of intraspecific variation assume that this approach avoids this problem.

This assumption is justified in some cases. Gill & Wolf had the best possible grounds for making that assumption about golden-winged sunbirds: the birds expressing two different social systems were not only from the same population, they were the same individuals. But this assumption is not always so well justified. In chapter 5 I have argued that one mechanism that would account for differences in social behavior is genetic differences between populations. Since populations are usually defined as genetically isolated subsets of a species, two populations may differ in the genetic basis for the observed variation in behavior. Thus, if the behavior observed does not bear out the predictions of the theory being tested it is still possible that the failure is due to phylogenetic inertia. In this case the inertia would be from a persisting genetic adjustment to a previous set of ecological circumstances which precludes adjustment to the present circumstances. This is a form of the 'ghost of determinants past' argument, but it is relevant because some ecological determinants can vary over short periods of time. Examples are: population density and hence intraspecific competition (including intruder pressure) prevalence of disease, predator pressure, population level of competitors, and presence of plant cover.

The impact of genetic differences in the predispositions of animals to interact in particular ways can be determined. An array of techniques is available to address this question, such as cross fostering and rearing in different physical environments. The fact that the variation occurs intraspecifically makes available another powerful technique from behavioral genetics: cross breeding.

If the results of such analyses were to show a significant degree of genetic determination of the observed differences in behavior then, as we have seen, the problems phylogenetic inertia poses for comparative interspecific socioecology are also posed when using intraspecific variation to test socioecological theory. On the other hand, genetic factors may be largely ruled out by such tests.

If the populations do not show evidence of genetic adaptation to their circumstances, then observed differences in their behavior must be due to some interaction with their circumstances. In such a case, selection has acted to produce a mechanism for flexibility rather than a single outcome. The interaction with the environment will take place through this mechanism. This mechanism reintroduces inertia in several ways.

8.6   ASSUMPTIONS ABOUT PHYLOGENETIC INERTIA AND MECHANISMS

Recall that we must expect two sorts of processes or mechanism in an instance of intraspecific variation in social systems. The first is a process that functions to assess the animal's circumstances and the alternative(s) available to it. The second mechanism is a process producing a change in social interactions and hence social systems. The first way that inertia is reintroduced is through the fact that these mechanisms are genetically based. While making a degree of flexibility possible they may also constrain the social system that might be expressed.

Here we encounter a major assumption in using intraspecific variation to test socioecological theory: that a shift to an alternative system will be a shift to the optimal system. This assumption will not always be correct. Consequently, when the observations do not conform to predictions it is not clear that the predictions have been tested. The hypothesis could correctly relate optimal behavior to the ecological determinants observed but not be confirmed because the behavior was not optimal. However, unless we know in what way and to what degree optimality is constrained, our hypothesis testing incorporates the doubtful assumption that animals expressing intraspecific variation always use the optimal system, selected without any constraints from a complete array that includes every possible alternative. The degree to which optimal adjustment could be achieved may be constrained in any of the several ways that are discussed in the chapters in which constraints are considered.

Krebs & Davies (1987) have pointed out that the expectations of optimal functioning are not realistic. Accordingly we could expect less than perfection but still be able to determine whether or not we have posed our question to nature in the right form and whether we are generally right. This is a reasonable approach, but it will often involve an *ad hoc* softening of the prediction made by the assumption of optimality.

8.7   CULTURAL INERTIA AND DEVELOPMENTAL MECHANISMS MAY CONSTRAIN OPTIMAL INTRASPECIFIC VARIATION

In addition to the genetic mechanisms, another mechanism that could constrain adjustment is cultural transmission of social systems and developmental mechanisms. Culturally transmitted social systems may not be strongly tested by their biological consequences (see also chapter 5). Other mechanisms would be developmental, including such things as sensitive period phenomena. One of the important implications of recognizing that intraspecific variation is produced by a mechanism is that the nature of the mechanism may influence a direct test of the theoretical predictions involved. It appears that whatever mechanism changes the social behavior of golden-winged sunbirds operates in the adult developmental stage. So far as we know, there is no stage in their lives when they cannot respond to changes in the ecological determinants of their social interactions.

But in other cases animals may initially have the potential to express several different behavior patterns, yet at some stage they become set and lose their potential for further flexibility. For example, we may discover that, in some cases, the particular social system observed depends on some process fixing it at a particular point in the development of each individual animal. If an animal's social pattern, say one that produces territoriality, becomes fixed at a point in development, its behavior could persist even though it is no longer optimal when circumstances change. An example might be individuals of a prey species developing a predisposition to be solitary in a habitat in which there was considerable cover from a dense community of woody plants. A fire could change that feature of their ecology in a few hours, making group living a more adaptive pattern. But these individuals might no longer have the potential plasticity to shift to the new pattern of behavior. In such a case the developmental stage at which the mechanism that produced social system variation operated would make the behavior of this population a poor test of socioecological predictions.

8.8   MAKING OPTIMAL USE OF INTRASPECIFIC VARIATION IN SOCIAL SYSTEMS

Analysis of the number and kind of assumptions involved in using intraspecific variation to test socioecological hypotheses is a bit daunting. We begin to wonder if there is any way to exploit the initially apparent advantages of avoiding the problem of phylogenetic inertia involved in interspecific comparisons. Happily, there are ways to exploit that difference. To take advantage of them, we must operate within the limits we have discussed, but even within those limits advantages remain. Let's consider some tactics.

Perhaps the best possible tactic is to get lucky. Most of the problems I have discussed will arise most forcefully when socioecological predictions fail. When they are confirmed the investigator is justified in asserting that the hypotheses has been confirmed. Of course, it will still be useful to keep the constraints outlined above in mind, and to be alert to the possibility of getting the right answer for the wrong reason.

Another tactic would be to use the developmental constraints noted above to our advantage. Suppose we find that the observed social system depends on some developmental process that fixes it at a particular point. Animals whose developmental history has determined they will express the social system usually observed in circumstances A (social system A') could be used to evaluate the fitness of the alternative social system B' (which is observed in circumstances B). Once their social behavior pattern had been fixed, they could be placed in circumstances B. By comparing the reproductive success of sets of animals manifesting each of the two social system alternatives in the one set of circumstances, the fitness of each of these alternatives in those circumstances could be compared.

Intraspecific variation has also made possible another related strategy for testing socioecological hypotheses that avoids merely assuming that the ecological variables studied are the determining variables. Instead of moving animals from one ecology to another we can switch the ecologies and observe the response of the animals. Ecologies can be switched by means of field experiments in which the investigator alters some proposed ecological determinant of social systems and watches for changes in the social system. A number of such manipulations are possible.

Some features of predator pressure can be manipulated by flying a trained raptor over the subjects (Kenward, 1978). The abundance and distribution of food can be varied as in a number of studies of the effect of nectar on the size of hummingbird territories (Norton *et al.*, 1982). The availability of storage sites can be manipulated (Stacey & Ligon, 1987). Demographic features such as sex ratios can be altered by adding or removing members of particular age and sex classes (Martin & Hannon, 1987). In this way the effect of habitat saturation on helping or sex ratios on polygamy, could be examined. Pleszczynska (1978) demonstrated a positive correlation between the amount of nest shade in the territory of a male savannah sparrow and the degree of polygyny expressed in that territory. Pleszczynska & Hansell (1980) then demonstrated that the correlated variable was a determinant, by producing polygyny through adding shade (strips of plastic) to territories with monogamous pairs and observing a shift to polygyny.

The spacing systems of mating male pronghorn antelope vary between territoriality and undefended home ranges (Byers & Kitchen, 1988). One likely determinant is the richness of resource patches. This hypothesis can be tested by creating rich resource patches via irrigation in a semi-arid area where the males are not territorial (Maher, in prep.).

While switching tactics or ecological determinants would provide the most compelling evidence that the behavior was at least more fit, an alternative approach would be to provide some evidence that the selection of the alternatives is the result of design, since evidence of design is a sort of prima facie evidence that a trait makes a contribution to fitness (Williams, 1966; Lewontin, 1979). One potential source of evidence of design is the mechanism by which the alternative social systems were produced. An analysis of the mechanism might show that it was especially evolved to produce the change, i.e., that it was an adaptation. In such cases there would be strong presumptive evidence that the alternatives were adaptive.

9

Practical importance of intraspecific variation in social systems

Intraspecific variation in social systems both creates problems for, and offers solutions to, people who manage animals. The problems arise when a management scheme depends on a species maintaining the same social system under different circumstances. The solutions arise when management schemes successfully predict and exploit a change in social systems to achieve some management end.

Most of the world's wild vertebrates live in rapidly changing circumstances. Many species are now endangered (usually because of human activities) and will not survive without active human intervention. To be effective, that intervention must be informed. One important piece of information is the ability to predict the kind of change in social systems that will occur in response to changes in circumstances. For certain management goals, that is essential. Perhaps the greatest promise that intraspecific variation offers for the solution of practical problems will be through the ability to predict the social system consequences of management manipulations or habitat alterations.

9.1 POPULATION DYNAMICS

Perhaps the most fundamental problem wildlife managers face is the prediction of population dynamics in a variety of situations. In populations limited by density dependent effects, an important determinant of population dynamics is the form competition takes. Contest competition tends to produce adequate resources for a relatively constant portion of a population. The bottom line is that breeding opportunities are restricted to a relatively constant portion of the population, making it rather stable. Scramble competition, in contrast, results in a more equal distribution of

183

resources in the population; so when resources are plentiful everyone has enough to reproduce and the population increases rapidly. In contrast, when resources are scarce, few have the resources to reproduce. Consequently a population in which resources are distributed by scramble competition fluctuates much more than a population in which resources are distributed by contest competition.

Since the kind of resource competition a population demonstrates is in part a function of the social system, variations in social systems within a population from territorial to undefended home ranges are likely to change the degree of stability in a population and increase its cyclic maximum while decreasing its cyclic minimum. The population dynamics of two populations of European rabbits (*Oryctolagus cuniculus*), one territorial and the other not, have been compared (Cowan & Garson, 1985); the features that could be ascertained followed the predicted trend. The differences in social systems observed were correlated with features of the ecology in the way predicted by socioecological theory (Cowan & Garson, 1985). The territorial population lived in an area where burrows and burrow sites were a limited resource. The burrows are patchily distributed and defended by females which effectively excluded other females from reproducing. The patchy distribution of reproducing females produced a resource that was defensible by males who were, in turn, territorial.

This means the manager may be able to predict population dynamics in part by determining the species' social system. It also means the manager may be able to manipulate the population dynamics of the species by manipulating its social system through changing its ecology.

A somewhat similar form of social impact on population dynamics is illustrated by Clutton-Brock & Albon's (1985) analysis of the reproductive consequences of large female mammals living in stable, closed groups. These authors pointed out that such groups are organized by dominance, with a greater share of the reproductive opportunities going to the most dominant individuals. They suggested this force operates constantly and stabilizes populations. However, the argument put forward by Clutton-Brock & Albon (1985) may only hold when groups are stable and closed. Populations of large mammals differ in whether females are in groups or solitary (e.g., Hirth, 1977) and whether groups are stable or unstable (Monfort-Brahm, 1975).

Impacts of social behavior on population dynamics seems to be greatest in species that naturally exist in relatively small populations, such as vertebrates in high trophic position (e.g., insectivores and carnivores).

Intraspecific variation is likely to occur in such species, and when it does it presents the greatest problems and possibilities to managers.

9.2   SMALL POPULATION MANAGEMENT

The management of small populations has become a major activity for conservation biology (Soule, 1986). The social systems of these small populations can have a major impact on goals such as the preservation of genetic diversity. One way in which the social system can affect the implementation of this goal is through the relationship of the mating system to the effective breeding population. The variation observed can be either a problem or a solution, depending on the management goals.

Most variation occurs for one of several reasons. The first is that resources vary. Among the most important resources are food and cover. Variation in both the absolute amount and the distribution of these two resources can have a profound effect on mating patterns. A second major factor is human disturbance. The most important forms of human disturbance are hunting and viewing or photographing animals. The form which is most important depends on the circumstances of the animals. Variations in the sex ratio of adults can have important effects on breeding systems. Group size may act as a determinant of mating systems and, thereby, of gene loss. Given that these variables can determine mating systems, management strategies to manipulate these systems, by varying their determinants, might be developed.

The greater the degree of polygyny a breeding system expresses the less genetic diversity is transmitted to the next generation. This is because the effective breeding population can be more a function of the breeding system than of the number of animals. For example, a population of 10 males and 10 females breeding monogamously has an effective breeding population of 20. However, the same population of males and females breeding in a system where one male does all the breeding will have an effective breeding population of only 3.54 (Frankel & Soule, 1981). (The reduction is this severe because half of all the genes in the next generation come from only one individual).

In fact polygyny is frequently an alternative to monogamy (see Chapter 3). Red foxes may express polygyny when the food resources within a territory are superabundant. It is easy to imagine a scenario in which attempts to sustain a small population could include supplementation of the food. Such supplementation could take a form that led to an increase in defensibility of food by a single male and thus increased the likelihood of a polygynous system. That would be a short term management step which would be contradictory to long term management goals.

9.3   HABITAT MANIPULATION AND INTRASPECIFIC SOCIAL SYSTEM VARIATION

Another factor that can change the social system of animals is habitat manipulation. White-tailed deer are always polygynous, but the degree of polygyny is likely to be a function of the distribution of the females. Their distribution is a function of habitat features (Hirth, 1977). Females in more open habitats are organized in groups rather than being solitary, and that organization makes it easier for individual males to control access to the females. This probably increases the degree of polygyny and decreases the size of the effective breeding population.

In some situations, females feed in territories held by males. The males in larger or richer territories have an advantage in breeding because females spend more time in a larger or richer territory. Circumstances reducing the cost of defending a larger or richer space can increase the potential of individual males to defend a better territory and so increase their breeding opportunities. For terrestrial vertebrates such situations include some boundary not requiring defense. Such a boundary may be the result of habitat feature or the distribution of a resource. Examples are the end of a peninsula or along a linear resource such as a river. Dippers in the end territories of a series along a river had larger territories and were polygynous (Price & Bock, 1973). Pronghorns at Wind Cave National Monument in South Dakota used uncrossable fences as part of their territorial boundary (Bromley, 1977). Because the fence constituted a boundary with no cost of defense, a larger area could be defended at the same cost as a smaller area. Since breeding success in territorial pronghorn antelope is a function of the amount of good forage within a male's territory (Kitchen, 1974), the degree of polygyny was likely to have increased in this situation and could be expected to increase in similar situations.

Since females are frequently the limiting resource in breeding systems, and since they suffer higher mortality than males in some systems, polyandry as an alternative to monogamy may produce an increase in the effective breeding population. An example of this would be California quail. Males virtually always outnumber females in a natural population, apparently because of higher mortality in females. These quail occasionally express serial polyandry (Francis, 1965). When they do, the effective breeding population is increased and genes of males which otherwise might not contribute to the next generation's gene pool are transmitted. In this case, the total output of young increases since the female produces more eggs and fledglings than she would otherwise, and the males may bear no reproductive cost of decreased output.

Cooperative polyandry as an alternative to monogamy has somewhat different trade-offs. Harris' hawks sometimes breed monogamously and at other times breed in cooperative polyandry (Mader, 1975b). Cooperative polyandry in this species may mean the exclusion of some females from breeding by the control of all suitable territories by breeding females. Even in such a case, polyandry will increase the genetic diversity of the next population; females that would have been excluded (had the population bred monogamously) will still be excluded under polyandry, but some of the males that would have been excluded will be represented.

9.4   MANAGING POPULATION SIZE

Another area where intraspecific variation in social systems has important implications is in the management of population size. Either increasing or decreasing a population's size is a common management goal. Social system change can frustrate these goals if it is not anticipated, but can facilitate them if it is.

A number of species facultatively express a breeding system with only one breeding pair in a social group. The other animals in the group act as helpers to the one breeding pair. In this social system the production of young per adult is typically much lower than it would be if all the adults were breeding. An attempt to reduce damage by a pest species by lowering the population size of this species (e.g., coyotes) would often lead to a change in social systems to breeding pairs without helpers. If that were to happen a large reduction in the population size might have little or no impact on the production of young. On the other hand, if an increase in population size were sought, one must anticipate that in the absence of dispersal a founder population of several breeding pairs would not continue to grow at its initial rate. A shift from pair breeding to communal breeding would develop as the population saturated its habitat. Recognition of this sort of social carrying capacity is important. It may constrain the population below the level at which basic resources such as food and nesting sites would allow it to grow.

Another impact of social systems on population levels can occur through the impact of the population's social system on female fecundity. Females breeding in a territorial system are subject to considerably less harassment than females breeding in a dominance system. To the degree that the harassment may influence their fecundity (e.g., Copeland, 1980), a shift from a territorial to a dominance system in the male spacing system will have an impact on the population's productivity.

A final impact of social system differences on productivity is the difference between monogamy and polygamy. In many species, mono-gamy confers the highest level of productivity per individual. In these species, any other breeding system decreases the level of care for each set of young and so decreases the productivity per breeding individual. Many species of birds are known to alternate between monogamy to polygyny under certain circumstances (see chapter 3). The population as a whole experiences loss of productivity.

Given these impacts of social system on population productivity, manipulating the variables influencing social systems will sometimes alter productivity. The percentage of animals breeding at any one time may be manipulated by varying the amount and distribution of resources. For example, if nest sites are created by management, it is important to recognize that clumped nest sites will be more easily defended by a single male and thus predispose the population to polygyny and a lower reproductive rate. If we want monogamy, we should create dispersed nest sites. Similarly, the distribution of food resources may influence the mating system of mammals by making it possible for an individual male to dominate sources of food as a resource females need and so give him disproportionate access to females.

Another way to manage productivity in a population is to modify the social system by eliminating or establishing territoriality. Since females are likely to be more fecund in a territorial system, the results of a change from dominance to territorial spacing is likely to produce an increase in productivity and vice versa. The likelihood of territoriality can be modified in at least two ways. The first is resource distribution. As I noted in discussing ecological determinants of intraspecific variation, a patchy distribution of food in economically defensible units increases the likeli-hood of a territorial system. On the other hand, disturbance by humans decreases the likelihood of a territorial system. Pronghorn antelope are a good example of the operation of both these factors. They are grassland browsers which evolved on the plains of North America. Although grassland itself is not patchily distributed on the plains, the forbs which the pronghorn seek within the grassland are often patchily distributed. When they are, pronghorn males are typically territorial and nearly all the breeding is done by the territory holders (Bromley 1969; Kitchen 1974). However, low levels of food availability or high levels of human disturbance by hunting will disrupt the territorial system (Kitchen, pers. comm.; Copeland, 1980). In the absence of territories, breeding takes place in large aggregations where breeding opportunities are distributed among the males via dominance relationships, and females are harassed much more than when breeding in the territorial system (Copeland, 1980; Byers & Kitchen, 1988).

9.5   CHANGE IN TRAITS FAVORED BY SELECTION

Different traits are favored by different social systems. If the spacing system is territorial and the breeding system polygynous, the type of animal favored will have traits promoting success in such a system. For example, shift to a dominance spacing system in ungulates may lead to a shift in the traits being passed on via the mating system. Territorial defense emphasizes attachment to the home range and often includes a high level of scent marking (Gosling, 1987). Marking activity will generally be of little use to a dominance-organized animal. It is not likely to be favored in a system in which non-marking animals would breed while the marking animal is scent-marking. Similarly, a dominance system combined with a polygynous system and female groups will tend to favor large males that dominate the breeding of the aggregated females. Changes in social group size could produce a change in the most advantageous male, since the large males are likely to be less effective in locating small, scattered females than smaller, more mobile males. If females are in groups where only one breeding-age male is likely to be present, selection may favor smaller males. They would also be favored in a situation where the smaller males with a less competitive strategy would have higher overwintering survival rates (Geist, 1971).

Given these relationships, it is possible to manage for the preferred behavioral and morphological types via manipulating the social system. In pronghorn antelope, for example, the set of traits underlying territoriality are favored by reducing human disturbance of the territorial bucks or by increasing rich food patches that promote territoriality. On the other hand the level of those traits can be reduced in the population by increasing human disturbance or reducing the richness and patchiness of the forage. To manage for the strongly polygynous system produced by strongly dimorphic, dominant individual males, one could buffer them against the natural catastrophes to which they are subject by providing them with supplemental food or shelter, reducing predator pressure, or using some other tactic to prevent their occasional catastrophic decline.

9.6   MANAGING SOCIAL BEHAVIOR AS A RESOURCE

Behavior is one of the most salient features of animals, and as such, is frequently a source of human interest in animals. Non-consumptive uses of animals, often emphasizing their behavior, is increasing rapidly (Clutton-Brock, 1990), but management for viewing behavior is not growing at the same rate. Some of the most interesting and appealing behavior occurs during social interactions. The territorial songs of birds are among the most common examples. Others are visual displays at territory boundaries, displays on leks, vocal communication among and between groups of wolves, coyotes, howler monkeys, and gibbons.

These displays are sometimes recognized by managers as a resource. A management plan for a Uganda kob population in Uganda, recognized the lekking display of the kob as an aesthetic resource to be managed and thus an economic resource to the people of Uganda (Buechner, 1974). The use of these behavior patterns as a resource may require management strategies to enhance or preserve their use. Relaxation of territoriality in pronghorns eliminates the territorial behavior that is potentially an important part of the experience of observing this species. In general, auditory and visual displays which function to get the attention of conspecifics are those most likely to get the attention of humans. Courtship and resource-defense behavior are likely to be dramatic and spectacular. Lekking, with its emphasis on competitive display, often creates a spectacular show. Several species alternate between lekking and some other form of breeding (Ugander kob, Leuthold, 1966; topi, Monfort- Brahm 1975; Duncan 1975; blue grouse (*Dendrogapus obscurus*), Blackford, 1958, 1963; Bendel, 1955; fallow deer (*Dama dama*), Clutton-Brock *et al.*, 1988). Where such shifts in behavior can be altered, their impact on non-consumptive uses of animals must be considered.

Vocalizations are used by territorial and dominance organized species. For example, male red deer (Clutton-Brock *et al.*, 1982), American bison (*Bison bison*) (Lott, 1979) and African lions (*Panthero leo*) (Schaller, 1972) roar. Wolves and coyotes howl. Such behavior occurs during particular social interactions; therefore, it can sometimes be managed.

Aggregation in general allows people to see many individuals of a species all at once, which may be desirable in the case of solitary animals. Many animals shift between flocking or schooling and being solitary and defending a territory as a function of certain environmental variables. Grizzly bears (*Ursus arctos*) are normally solitary, but they form large aggregations at the mouths of rivers in Alaska when the the salmon are running up the river to spawn. This behavioral shift provides an exceptional opportunity to see a great show. This aggregation occurs as a function of natural processes. For a number of years, the National Park Service in Yellowstone National Park, Wyoming encouraged the same sort of grizzly bear aggregations for visitor benefit by using garbage as the attraction (Craighead, 1979). I do not recommend this practice, but it demonstrates the possibilities for powerful changes in behavior.

Changes in behavior constituting a public resource will often be managed by manipulating the causes of alternative expressions of that behavior. What causes changes in behavior is not always clear, because what produces the behavior of interest is not always clear. We do not always know why animals lek in some circumstances and not in others. A prominent theory is that males lek in areas that females favor for some other reason (Bradbury, 1981; Gosling, 1986; Clutton-Brock, 1990). If that is so, management for lekking would consist of managing the resources that attract females to a particular place, such as areas with a high food resource. Alternatively, there might be areas of lowered predation risk, such as an area with fewer predators or one in which prey have a greater opportunity to detect or escape predators.

The sources of territorial behavior are more frequently known and thus are more manipulable. Territorial behavior that functions to enhance foraging may be produced by abundant resources within an economically defensible range. According to this model, too many or too few resources are likely to lead to relaxation of territoriality. Factors that influence the defense of foraging territories are the foods' distribution in space and the presence and activity of predators. Wintering sanderlings are a good example of the impact of these variables on the defense of foraging territories (Myers *et al.*, 1979a,b). A population disturbed regularly by a lot of human activity might be disrupted in its territorial behavior in much the same way.

Management of these behavior patterns requires manipulating the variables determining their appearance. Sometimes the amount of food available can be manipulated. The food available to a population can be supplemented in various ways. By modifying the natural production system in the area through fertilizing or irrigating the plant community, food production can be increased. Sometimes the distribution of resources can be varied. Food, cover, minerals and water can all be supplied in varying degrees of patchiness. The degree of patchiness of these resources is likely to influence the probability of territorial defense. This is particularly true for social systems organized around access to primary resources by the consumer. This is also true, to a degree, of social systems organized to distribute mating opportunities as a resource. In most such systems, females are the resource, and their distribution is influenced by the distribution of the resources they use directly as consumers (Wrangham, 1986).

9.7   MANAGING HUMAN DISTURBANCE

The impact of human disturbance on social systems can, at least in theory, be readily managed. In practice, however, that can prove difficult. As noted earlier, Copeland (1980) observed adverse effects of sport hunting on pronghorn territorial behavior. He recommended delaying the hunting season a few weeks until the breeding season had passed and the territories were abandoned. His recommendation was, at least initially, rejected on the ground that hunters had grown accustomed to planning their hunt for a particular time and would not want to change (Hornocker, pers. comm.). Deblinger & Alldredge (1989) also observed a very similar effect of hunting on a pronghorn breeding system. They endorsed Copeland's recommendation as being the most practical way to protect the genetic outcomes favored by undisturbed natural selection.

Predation has a strong impact on social systems and sometimes can be modified either by increasing or decreasing predator density. Such manipulations could change the social systems of both predator and prey alike. Many programs reduce predator abundance, and a few reintroduce predators (e.g., wolves) into areas from which they have been extirpated (Mech, 1970). Many issues determine such a decision, but the impact of such management on the social system of the prey species has not usually been one of them. It should be an issue in future decisions.

9.8   CONCLUSION

At the beginning of this chapter I noted that intraspecific variation in social systems creates management problems and offers management solutions. Examples in the previous pages illustrate both problems and solutions. The use of a recently appreciated phenomenon as a management and conservation tool is a little daunting in some ways. We are handicapped by the lack of a full understanding of the phenomenon. In particular, we have little real grasp of the mechanisms that produce particular alternatives, and this constrains our ability to predict the exact consequence of specific strategies.

But we do know what circumstances are likely to produce particular outcomes, and conservation decisions will be better made with partial knowledge than complete ignorance of their impact on social systems. With that knowledge comes the responsibility to make the contribution we can now, while we work toward the increased understanding that will allow us to make an even greater contribution in the future.

References

Adams, N. R., Hearnshaw, H. & Oldman, C. M. (1981). Abnormal function of the corpus luteum in some ewes with phytoestrogenic infertility. *Australian Journal of Biological Science*, **34**, 61–5.

Ahlen, I. & Andersson, A. (1970). Breeding ecology of an eider population on Spitsbergen. *Ornis Scandinavica*, **1**, 83–106.

Alatalo, R. V., Gustafsson, L. & Lundberg, A. (1986). Do females prefer older males in polygynous bird species? *American Naturalist*, **127**, 241–5.

Alatalo, R. V. & Lundberg, A. (1984). Polyterritorial polygyny in the pied flycatcher *Ficedula hypoleuca* – evidence for the deception hypothesis. *Annals Zoologica Fennici*, **21**, 217–28.

Alcock, J. (1984). *Animal Behavior: An Evolutionary Approach*. Sunderland, MA: Sinauer Associates.

Alexander, R. D. (1974). The evolution of social behavior. *Annual Review of Ecology and Systematics*, **5**, 325–83.

Altenburg, W., Daan, S., Starkenburg, J. & Zijlstra, M. (1982). Polygamy in the marsh harrier, *Circus aeruginosus*: individual variation in hunting performance and number of mates. *Behaviour*, **79**, 272–312.

Altmann, S. A. & Altmann, J. (1979). Demographic constraints on behavior and social organization. In *Primate Ecology and Human Origins: Ecological Influences on Social Organization*, ed. I. Bernstein & E. O. Smith, pp. 47–63. New York: Garland STPM Press.

Andelt, W. F. (1985). Behavioral ecology of coyotes in south Texas. *Wildlife Monographs*, **94**, 1–45.

Anderson, P. K. (1961). Density, social structure, and nonsocial environment in house mouse populations and the implications for regulation of numbers. *Transactions New York Academy of Science*, **23**, 447–51.

Anderson, P. K. & Hill, J. L. (1965). *Mus musculus*: experimental induction of territory formation. *Science*, **148**, 1753–5.

Andersson, M. (1984). Brood parasitism within species. In *Strategies of Exploitation and Parasitism*, ed. C. J. Barnard, pp. 195–227. London: Croom Helm.

Andersson, M. & Gotmark, F. (1980). Social organization and foraging ecology in the arctic skua *Stercorarius parasiticus*: a test of the food defendability hypotheses. *Oikos*, **35**, 63–71.

Ankney, C. D. & Scott, D. M. (1982). On the mating system of brown-headed cowbirds. *Wilson Bulletin*, **94**, 260–8.

Armitage, K. B. (1977). Social variety in the yellow-bellied marmot: a population–behavioural system. *Animal Behavior*, **25**, 585–93.

(1988). Resources and social organization of ground-dwelling squirrels. In *The Ecology of Social Behavior*, ed. C. M. Slobodchikoff, pp. 131–55. San Diego: Academic Press.

Armitage, K. B. & Downhower, J. F. (1974). Demography of yellow-bellied marmot populations. *Ecology*, **55**, 1233–45.

Austad, S. N. & Rabenold, K. N. (1985). Reproductive enhancement by helpers and an experimental inquiry into its mechanism in the bicolored wren. *Behavioural Ecology and Sociobiology*, **17**, 19–27.

Avery, M. L. (1982). Nesting biology, seasonality, and mating system of Malaysian fantail warblers. *Condor*, **84**, 106–9.

Bacon, P. J. (1980). Status and dynamics of a mute swan population near Oxford between 1976 and 1978. *Wildfowl*, **31**, 37–50.

Balfour, E. & Cadbury, C. J. (1979). Polygyny, spacing and sex ratio among hen harriers *Circus cyaneus* in Orkney, Scotland. *Ornis Scandinavica*, **10**, 133–41.

Balph, D. F. & Balph, M. H. (1979). Behavioral flexibility of pine siskins in mixed species foraging groups. *Condor*, **81**, 211–2.

Balph, D. F., Innis, G. S. & Balph, M. H. (1980). Kin selection in Rio Grande turkeys: a critical assessment. *Auk*, **97**, 854–60.

Barlow, G. W. (1974). Extraspecific imposition of social grouping among surgeonfishes (Pisces: Acanthuridae). *Journal of Zoology, London*, **174**, 333–40.

Barnett, S. A. (1958). An analysis of social behaviour in wild rats. *Proceedings of the Zoological Society of London*, **130**, 107–52.

Barres, R. H., Moore, A. U. & Pond, W. G. (1970). Behavioural abnormalities in young adult pigs caused by malnutrition in early life. *Journal of Nutrition*, **100**, 149.

Barrette, C. (1988). Causal analysis in behavioural ecology. *Animal Behaviour*, **36**, 310.

Bateson, P. (1987). Biological approaches to the study of behavioural development. *International Journal of Behavioral Development*, **10**, 1–22.

Beason, R. C. & Trout, L. L. (1984). Cooperative breeding in the bobolink. *Wilson Bulletin*, **96**, 709–10.

Bednarz, J. C. (1987). Pair and group reproductive success, polyandry, and cooperative breeding in Harris' hawks. *Auk*, **104**, 393–404.

(1988). Cooperative hunting in Harris' hawks (*Parabuteo unicinctus*). *Science*, **239**, 1525–7.

Bednarz, J. C. & Ligon, J. D. (1988). A study of the ecological bases of cooperative breeding in the Harris' hawk. *Ecology*, **69**, 1176–87.

Beissinger, S. R. (1986). Demography, environmental uncertainty, and the evolution of mate desertion in the snail kite. *Ecology*, **67**, 1445–59.

Bekoff, M. (1978). Behavioral development in coyotes and eastern coyotes. In

Coyotes: Biology, Behavior, and Management, ed. M. Bekoff, pp. 97–126. New York: Academic Press.

Bekoff, M., Daniels, T. J. & Gittleman, J. L. (1984). Life history patterns and the comparative social ecology of carnivores. *Annual Review of Ecology and Systematics*, **15**, 191–232.

Bekoff, M. & Wells, M. C. (1980). The social ecology of coyotes. *Scientific American*, **242**, 130–51.

Bendell, J. F. (1955). Age, breeding behavior and migration of the sooty grouse (*Dendgapus obscurus fulignosis*) (Ridgeway). *Transactions of the Twentieth North American Wildlife Conference*, 367–81.

Bennets, H. W., Underwood, E. J. & Shier, F. L. (1946). A specific problem of sheep on subterranean clover pastures in western Australia. *Australian Veterinary Journal*, **22**, 2–12.

Berger, J. (1979). Social ontogeny and behavioural diversity: consequences for bighorn sheep *Ovis canadensis* inhabiting desert and mountain environments. *Journal of Zoology, London*, **188**, 251–66.

(1988). Social systems, resources and phyogenetic inertia: an experimental test and its limitations. In *The Ecology of Social Behavior*, ed. C. M. Slobodchikoff, pp. 157–86. San Diego: Academic Press.

Berger, P. J., Sanders, E. H., Gardner, P. D. & Negus, N. C. (1977). Phenolic plant compounds functioning as reproductive inhibitors in *Microtus montanus*. *Science*, **195**, 575–7.

Bernstein, I. S. (1976). Dominance, aggression and reproduction in primate societies. *Journal of Theoretical Biology*, **60**, 459–72.

Berry, K. H. (1974). The ecology and social behavior of the chuckwalla, *Sauromalus obesus obesus* Baird. *University of California Publications in Zoology*, **101**.

Bertram, B. G. R. (1978). Living in groups: predators and prey. In *Behavioural Ecology*, ed. J. R. Krebs & N. B. Davies, pp. 64–96. Sunderland, MA: Sinauer Associates.

Birkhead, T. R. & Clarkson, K. (1985). Ceremonial gatherings of the magpie *Pica pica*: territory probing and acquisition. *Behaviour*, **94**, 324–32.

Birkhead, T. R., Eden, S. F., Clarkson, K., Goodburn, S. F. & Pellatt, J. (1985). Social organisation of a population of magpies *Pica pica*. *Ardea*, **74**, 59–68.

Blackford, J. L. (1958). Territoriality and breeding behavior of a population of blue grouse in Montana. *Condor*, **60**, 145–58.

(1963). Further observations on the breeding behavior of a blue grouse population in Montana. *Condor*, **65**, 485–516.

Bleich, V. C. & Schwartz, O. A. (1975). Observations on the home range of the desert woodrat, *Neotoma lepida intermedia*. *Journal of Mammalogy*, **56**, 518–9.

Bloch, D. (1970). Knopsvanen (*Cygnus olor*) some kolonifugl i Danmark. *Danske Ornitologisk forenings Tidsskrift*, **64**, 152–62.

Blockstein, D. E. (1986). Nesting trios of mourning doves. *Wilson Bulletin*, **98**, 309–11.

Bolles, R. C. (1970). Species-specific defense reactions and avoidance learning. *Psychological Review*, **77**, 32–48.

(1975). *Learning Theory*. New York: Holt, Rinehardt & Winston.

Bollinger, E. K., Gavin, T. A., Hibbard, C. J. & Wootton, J. T. (1986). Two male bobolinks feed young at the same nest. *Wilson Bulletin*, **98**, 154–6.

Boness, D. J., Bowen, W. D. & Oftedal, O. T. (1988). Evidence of polygyny from spatial patterns of hooded seals (*Cystophora cristata*). *Canadian Journal of Zoology*, **66**, 703–6.

Bonner, J. T. (1980). *The Evolution of Culture in Animals*. Princeton, NJ: Princeton University Press.

Botsford, L. W., Wainwright, T. C., Smith, J. T., Mastrup, S. & Lott, D. F. (1988). Population dynamics of California quail related to meteorological conditions. *Journal of Wildlife Management*, **52**, 469–77.

Bovet, D. (1977). Strain differences in learning in the mouse. In *Genetics, Environment and Intelligence*, ed. E. A. Oliverio, pp. 79–92. Amsterdam: North Holland Publishing Co.

Bowen, W. D. (1981). Variation in coyote social organization: the influence of prey size. *Canadian Journal of Zoology*, **59**, 639–52.

Bowyer, R. T. (1987). Coyote group size relative to predation on mule deer. *Mammalia*, **51**, 515–26.

Boyd, R. & Richerson, P. J. (1985). *Culture and the Evolutionary Process*. Chicago: University of Chicago Press.

Bradbury, J. (1981). The evolution of leks. In *Natural Selection and Social Behavior*, ed. R. D. Alexander & D. W. Tinkle, pp. 138–69. New York: Chiron Press.

Bradbury, J. T. & White, D. E. (1954). Estrogens and related substances in plants. *Vitamins and Hormones*, **12**, 207–33.

Bradbury, J. W. & Gibson, R. M. (1983). Leks and mate choice. In *Mate Choice*, ed. P. P. G. Bateson, pp. 107–38. Cambridge: Cambridge University Press.

Bragg, A. N. (1955). In quest of the spadefoots. *New Mexico Quarterly*, **25**, 345–57.

Braithwaite, L. W. (1981). Ecological studies of the black swan III. Behaviour and social organization. *Australian Wildlife Research*, **8**, 135–46.

Brakhage, G. K. (1965). Biology and behavior of tub-nesting Canada geese. *Journal of Wildlife Management*, **29**, 751–71.

Breitwisch, R., Ritter, R. C. & Zaias, J. (1986). Parental behavior of a bigamous male northern mockingbird. *Auk*, **103**, 424–7.

Breland, K. & Breland, M. (1967). The misbehavior of organisms. *American Psychologist*, **16**, 681–4.

Briskie, J. V. & Sealy, S. G. (1987). Polygyny and double-brooding in the least flycatcher. *Wilson Bulletin*, **99**, 492–4.

Bromley, P. T. (1969). Territoriality in pronghorn bucks on the National Bison Range, Moiese, Montana. *Journal of Mammalogy*, **50**, 281–9.

(1977). Aspects of the behavioral ecology and sociobiology of the pronghorn (*Antilocapra americana*). Ph.D. Dissertation. University of Calgary, Alberta.

Bromley, P. T. & Kitchen, D. W. (1974). Courtship in the pronghorn (*Antilocapra americana*). In *The Behaviour of Ungulates and its Relation to Management*, ed. V. Geist & F. R. Walther. Morges, Switzerland: IUCN.

Bronson, F. H. (1979). The reproductive ecology of the house mouse. *Quarterly Review of Biology*, **54**, 265–99.

Brown, C. R. (1975). Polygymy in the purple martin. *Auk*, **92**, 602–4.

(1979). Territoriality in the purple martin. *Wilson Bulletin*, **91**, 583–91.

Brown, J. L. (1964). The evolution of diversity in avian territorial systems. *Wilson Bulletin*, **76**, 160–9.

(1978). Avian communal breeding systems. *Annual Review of Ecology and Systematics*, **9**, 123–55.

(1987). *Helping and Communal Breeding in Birds*. Princeton, NJ: Princeton University Press.

Brown, J. L. & Balda, R. P. (1977). The relationship of habitat quality to group size in Hall's babbler (*Pomatostomus halli*). *Condor*, **79**, 312–20.

Brown, J. L., Dow, D. D., Brown, E. R. & Brown, S. D. (1978). Effects of helpers on feeding of nestlings in the grey-crowned babbler (*Pomatostomus temporalis*). *Behavioural Ecology and Sociobiology*, **4**, 43–59.

(1983). Socioecology of the grey-crowned babbler: population structure, unit size and vegetation correlates. *Behavioral Ecology and Sociobiology*, **13**, 115–24.

Browne, P. M., Duffus, D. A. & Boychuk, R. W. (1983). High nesting density of ducks on an island in Saskatchewan. *Canadian Field-Naturalist*, **97**, 453–4.

Brunton, D. H. (1988). Sequential polyandry by a female killdeer. *Wilson Bulletin*, **100**, 670–2.

Bryson, R. A. (1974). A perspective on climatic change. *Science,* **184**, 753–60.

(1980). Ancient climes on the Great Plains. *Natural History*, **89**, 64–73.

Bryson, R. A. & Murray, T. J. (1977). *Climates of Hunger*. Madison: University of Wisconsin Press.

Buckman, N. S. & Ogden, J. C. (1973). Territorial behavior of the striped parrotfish *Scarus croicensis* Bloch (Scaridae). *Ecology*, **54**, 1377–82.

Buechner, H. K. (1974). Implications of social behavior in the management of Uganda kob. In *The Behaviour of Ungulates and its Relation to Management*, ed. V. Geist & F. E. Walther, pp. 853–70. Morges, Switzerland: IUCN.

Bull, C. J. & McInerney, J. E. (1974). Behavior of juvenile coho salmon (*Onchorhynchus kisutch*) exposed to Sumithon (fenitrothion, an organophosphate insecticide). *Journal of the Fisheries Research Board of Canada*, **31**, 1867–72.

Bunni, M. K. (1959). *The Killdeer in the Breeding Season*. Ph.D. thesis, University of Michigan.

Burger, J. (1974). Breeding biology and ecology of the brown-hooded gull in Argentina. *Auk*, **91**, 601–13.

Burgess, J. W. & Coss, R.G. (1981). Short-term juvenile crowding arrests the developmental formation of dendritic spines on tectal interneurons in jewel fish. *Developmental Psychobiology*, **14**, 389–96.

Burley, M. (1986). Sexual selection for aesthetic traits in species with biparental care. *American Naturalist*, **127**, 415–45.

Busher, P. E., Warner, R. J. & Jenkins, S. H. (1983). Population density, colony composition, and local movements in two Sierra Nevadan beaver populations. *Journal of Mammalogy*, **64**, 314–18.

Byers, J. A. & Kitchen, D. W. (1988). Mating system shift in a pronghorn population. *Behavioral Ecology and Sociobiology*, **22**, 355–60.

Caldwell, G. S. (1986). Predation as a selective force on foraging herons: effects of plumage color and flocking. *Auk*, **103**, 494–505.

Camenzind, F. J. (1978). Behavioral ecology of coyotes on the National Elk Refuge, Jackson, Wyoming. In *Coyotes: Biology, Behavior and Management*, ed. M. Bekoff, pp. 267–94. New York: Academic Press.

Campagna, C., Le Boeuf, B. J., & Cappozzo, H. L. (1988). Group raids: a mating strategy of male southern sea lions. *Behaviour*, **105**, 224–49.

Caraco, T. (1979a). Time budgeting and group size: a theory. *Ecology*, **60**, 611–17.

(1979b). Time budgeting and groups size: a test of theory. *Ecology*, **60**, 618–27.

Caraco, T. & Wolf, L. L. (1975). Ecological determinants of group size of foraging lions. *American Naturalist*, **109**, 343–52.

Carey, M. & Nolan, V. Jr. (1975). Polygyny in indigo buntings: a hypothesis tested. *Science*, **190**, 1296–7.

(1979). Population dynamics of indigo buntings and the evolution of avian polygyny. *Evolution*, **33**, 1180–92.

Carlsson, B.-G., Hornfeldt, B. & Lofgren, O. (1987). Bigamy in Tengmalm's owl *Aegolius funereus*: effect of mating strategy on breeding success. *Ornis Scandinavica*, **18**, 237–43.

Caro, T. M. & Bateson, P. (1986). Organization and ontogeny of alternative tactics. *Animal Behavior*, **34**, 1483–99.

Caro, T. M. & Collins, D. A. (1986). Male cheetahs of the Serengeti. *National Geographic Research*, **2**, 75–86.

(1987). Male cheetah social organization and territoriality. *Ethology*, **74**, 52–64.

Carpenter, C. R. (1940). A field study in Siam of the behavior and social relations of the gibbon (*Hylobates lar*). *Comparative Psychology Monographs*, **16**, 1–212.

Carpenter, F. L. & MacMillen, R. E. (1976). Threshold model of feeding territoriality and test with a Hawaiian honeycreeper. *Science*, **194**, 639–42.

Carrick, R, (1963). Ecological significance of territory in the Australian magpie. *Proceedings of the XIII International Ornithological Congress*, 740–53.

Cartar, R. V. & Lyon, B. E. (1988). The mating system of the buff-breasted sandpiper: lekking and resource defense polygyny. *Ornis Scandinavica*, **19**, 74–6.

Chadwick, D. H. (1983). *A Beast the Color of Winter*. San Francisco: Sierra Club Books.

Chamberlin, M. L. (1977). Observations on the red-necked grebe nesting in Michigan. *Wilson Bulletin*, **89**, 33–46.

Charnov, E. L. (1981). Kin selection and helpers at the nest: effects of paternity and biparental care. *Animal Behaviour*, **29**, 631–2.

Chepko-Sade, B. D. & Halpin, Z.T. ed. (1987). *Mammalian dispersal patterns*. Chicago: University of Chicago Press.

Christie, M. H. & Barfield, R. J. (1979). Effects of castration and home cage residency on aggressive behavior in rats. *Hormones and Behavior*, **13**, 85–91.

Clavijo, I. E. (1983). Pair Spawning and formation of a lek-like mating system in the parrotfish *Scarus vetula*. *Copeia*, 1983, 253–6.

Clemens, L. G. & Glaude, B. A. (1978). Femnine sexual behavior in rats enhanced by prenatal inhibition of androgen aromatization. *Hormones and Behavior*, **11**, 190–201.

Clutton-Brock, T. H. (1990). Mammalian mating systems. *Proceedings of the Royal Society, London*, B. (In press.)

Clutton-Brock, T. H. & Albon, S. D. (1985). The roaring of red deer and the evolution of honest advertisement. *Behaviour*, **69**, 145–70.

Clutton-Brock, T. H. & Albon, S. D. & Guinness, F. E. (1982). *Red Deer: the Ecology of Two Sexes*. Chicago: University of Chicago Press.

Clutton-Brock, T. H., Green, D., Hiraiwa-Hasegawa, M & Albon, S. D. (1988). Passing the buck: resource defence, lek breeding and mate choice in fallow deer. *Behavioral Ecology and Sociobiology*, **23**, 281–96.

Clutton-Brock, T. H. & Harvey, P. H. (1977). Primate ecology and social organization. *Joural of Zoology, London*, **183**, 1–39.

   (1984). Comparative approaches to investigating adaptation. In *Behavioural Ecology: An Evolutionary Approach*, ed. J. R. Krebs & N. B Davies, pp. 7–29. Oxford: Blackwell Scientific Publications.

Cole, K. S. & Noakes, D. L. G. (1980). Development of early social behaviour of rainbow trout, *Salmo gairdneri* (Pisces, Salmonidae). *Behavioural Processes*, **5**, 97–112.

Collias, N. E. (1950). Some variations in grouping and dominance patterns among birds and mammals. *Zoologica*, **35**, 97–119.

Colwell, M. A. (1986). The first documented case of polyandry for Wilson's phalarope (*Phalaropus tricolor*). *Auk*, **103**, 611–12.

Colwell, M. A. & Oring, L. W. (1988). Variable female mating tactics in a sex-role-reversed shorebird, Wilson's phalarope (*Phalaropus tricolor*). *National Geographic Research*, **4**, 408–15.

Connors, P. G., Myers, J. P., Connors, C. S. W. & Pitelka, F. A. (1981). Interhabitat movement by sanderlings in relation to foraging profitability and the tidal cycle. *Auk*, **98**, 49–64.

Conover, M. R., Miller, D. E. & Hunt, G. L. Jr. (1979). Female-female pairs and other unusual reproductive associations in ring-billed and California gulls. *Auk*, **96**, 6–9.

Copeland, G. L. (1980). Antelope buck breeding behavior, habitat selection and hunting impact. *Idaho Department of Fish and Game Wildlife Bulletin*, **8**, 1–45.

Cords, M. (1984). Mating patterns and social structure in redtail monkeys (*Cercopithecus ascanius*). *Zeitschrift für Tierpsychologie*, **64**, 313–29.

Coss, R. G. & Burgess, J. W. (1981). Jewel fish retain juvenile schooling pattern after crowded development. *Developmental Psychobiology*, **14**, 451–7.

Cowan, D. P. & Bell, D. J. (1986). Leporid social behaviour and social organization. *Mammal Review*, **16**, 169–79.

Cowan, D. P. & Garson, P. J. (1985). Variations in the social structure of rabbit populations: causes and demographic consequences. In *Behavioural Ecology: Ecological Consequences of Adaptive Behaviour*, ed. R. M. Sibly & R. H. Smith, pp. 537–55. Oxford: Blackwell Scientific Publications.

Cowley, E. (1983). Multi-brooding and mate infidelity in the sand martin. *Bird Study*, **30**, 1–7.

Craig, A. J. F. K. (1987). Co-operative breeding the pied starling. *Ostrich*, **58**, 176–80.

Craig, J. L. (1979). Habitat variation in the social organization of a communal gallinule, the pukeko, *Porphyrio porphyrio melanotus*. *Behavioural Ecology and Sociobiology*, **5**, 331–58.

(1980). Breeding success of a communal gallinule. *Behavioural Ecology and Sociobiology*, **6**, 289–95.

(1984). Are communal pukeko caught in the prisoner's dilemma? *Behavioural Ecology and Sociobiology*, **14**, 147–50.

Craighead, F. C. Jr. (1979). *Track of the Grizzly*. San Francisco: Sierra Club Books.

Crawford, R.D. (1977). Polygynous breeding of short-billed marsh wrens. *Auk*, **94**, 359–62.

Crick, H. Q. P. & Fry, C. H. (1986). Effects of helpers on parental condition in red-throated bee-eaters (*Merops bullocki*). *Journal of Animal Ecology*, **55**, 893–905.

Crome, F. H. J. & Brown, H. E. (1979). Notes on social organization and breeding of the orange-footed scrubfowl *Megapodius reinwardt*. *Emu*, **79**, 111–19.

Crook, J. H. (1961). The fodies (Ploceinae) of the Seychelles Islands. *Ibis*, **103**, 517–48.

(1965). The adaptive significance of avian social organizations. *Symposium of the Zoological Society of London*, **14**, 181–218.

(1970). The socio-ecology of primates. In *Social Behaviour in Birds and Mammals*, ed. J. H.Crook, pp. 103–66. London: Academic Press.

(1989). Socioecological paradigms, evolution and history: perspectives for the 1990s. In *Comparative Socioecology: the Behavioural Ecology of Humans and Other Animals*, ed. V. Standen & R. Foley, pp. 1–35. Oxford, Blackwell Scientific Publications.

Crook, J. H. & Gartlan, J. S. (1966). Evolution of primate societies. *Nature*, **210**, 1200–3.

Crow, J. F. & Kimura, M. (1970). *An Introduction to Population Genetics Theory*. New York: Harper & Row.

Crowcroft, P. (1955). Territoriality in wild house mice, *Mus musculus L. Journal of Mammalogy*, **36**, 299–301.

Curio, E. (1975). The functional organization of anti-predator behaviour in the pied flycatcher: a study of avian visual perception. *Animal Behavior*, **23**, 1–115.

(1978). The adaptive significance of avian mobbing. *Zeitschrift für Tierpsychologie*, **48**, 175–83.

Curry, R. L. (1988). Influence of kinship on helping behavior in Galapagos mockingbirds. *Behavioral Ecology and Sociobiology*, **22**, 141–52.

Darling, F. F. (1937). *A Herd of Red Deer*. London: Oxford University Press.

Darwin, C. R. (1859). *The Origin of Species*. London: John Murray.

DaSilva, J. & Terhune, J. M. (1988). Harbour seal grouping as an anti-predator strategy. *Animal Behavior*, **36**, 1309–16.

Davies, N. B. (1976). Food, flocking and territorial behaviour of the pied wagtail (*Motacilla alba yarrellii* Gould) in winter. *Journal of Animal Ecology*, **45**, 235–54.

Davies, N. B. (1978). Ecological questions about territorial behaviour. In *Behavioural Ecology*, ed. J. R. Krebs & N. B. Davies, pp. 317–50. Sunderland, MA: Sinauer Associates, Inc.

(1989). Sexual conflict and the polygyny threshold. *Animal Behavior*, **38**, 226–234.

Davies, N. B. & Houston, A. I. (1983). Time allocation between territories and flocks and owner-satellite conflict in foraging pied wagtails, *Motacilla alba*. *Journal of Animal Ecology*, **52**, 621–34.

(1986). Reproductive success of dunnocks, *Prunella modularis*, in a variable mating system. II. Conflicts of interest among breeding adults. *Journal of Animal Ecology*, **55**, 139–54.

Davies, N. B. & Lundberg, A. (1984). Food distribution and a variable mating system in the dunnock, *Prunella modularis*. *Journal of Animal Ecology*, **53**, 895–912.

Davis, D. E. (1941). The relation of abundance to territorialism in tropical birds. *Bird-Banding*, **12**, 93–7.

(1958). The role of density in aggressive behaviour of house mice. *Animal Behaviour*, **6**, 207–10.

Dawkins, R. (1976). *The Selfish Gene*. Oxford: Oxford University Press.

De Ghett, V. J. (1975). A factor influencing aggression in adult mice: witnessing aggression when young. *Behavioural Biology*, **13**, 291–300.

Deblinger, R. D. & Alldredge, A. W. (1989). Management implications of variations in pronghorn social behavior. *Wildlife Society Bulletin*, **17**, 82–7.

Decoux, J. P. (1982). Les particularites demographiques et sociecologiques du coliou strie dans le nord-est du Gabon. I. Donees d'observation. *Review of Ecology*, **36**, 37–78.

(1983). Les particularites demographiques et sociecologiques du coliou strie dans le nord-est du Gabon. II. Strategies adaptatives de l'espece. *Review of Ecology*, **37**, 219–40.

DellaSala, D. A. (1985). The yellow warbler in southeastern Michigan: factors affecting its productivity. *Jack-Pine Warbler*, **63**, 10 pp.

(1986). Polygyny in the yellow warbler. *Wilson Bulletin*, **98**, 152–4.

DeMan, E. & Peeke, H. V. S. (1982). Dietary ferulic acid, biochanin A, and the inhibition of reproductive function in Japanese quail (*Coturnix coturnix*). *Pharmacology Biochemistry and Behavior*, **17**, 405–11.

Dewar, J. M. (1937). Ménage a trois in the mute swan. *British Birds*, **30**, 178–9.

Dewsbury, D. A. (1982). Dominance rank, copulatory behavior, and differential reproduction. *The Quarterly Review of Biology*, **57**, 135–59.

Dhondt, A. A. (1987a). Reproduction and survival of polygynous and monogamous blue tit *Parus caeruleus*. *Ibis*, **129**, 327–34.

(1987b). Polygynous blue tits and monogamous great tits: does the polygyny-threshold model hold? *American Naturalist*, **129**, 213–20.

Dickinson, A. (1980). *Contemporary Animal Learning Theory*. Cambridge: Cambridge University Press.

Dolhinow, P. (1977). Comment on 'Infanticide as a primate reproductive strategy' by Hrdy, S. B. *American Scientist*, **65**, 40–9.

Dow, D. D. (1979a). Communally breeding Australian birds with an analysis of distributional and environmental factors. *Emu*, **80**, 121–40.

(1979b). The influence of nests on the social behaviour of males in *Manorina melanocephala*, a communally breeding honeyeater. *Emu*, **79**, 71–83.

Dowsett-Lemaire, F. (1979). The sexual bond in the marsh warbler *Acrocephalus palustris*. *Le Gerfaut*, **69**, 3–12.

Duffy, A. M. Jr. (1982). Movements and activities of radio-tracked brown-headed cowbirds. *Auk*, **99**, 316–27.

Duffy, D. C. (1980). *Comparative reproductive behavior and population regulation of seabirds of the Peruvian coastal current*. Ph.D. Thesis, Princeton University, Princeton, New Jersey.

Dunbar, R. I. M. (1982). Intraspecific variations in mating strategy. *Perspectives in Ethology*, **5**. 385–431.

(1988). *Primate Social Systems*. Ithaca: Cornell University Press.

Duncan, P. (1975). *Topi and Their Food Supply*. Ph.D. Dissertation. University of Nairobi, Nairobi, Kenya.

Earle, R. A. (1987). A case of bigamy in the redbreasted swallow *Hirundo semirufa*. *South African Journal of Zoology*, **22**, 325–6.

Earle, R. A. & Herholdt, J. J. (1986). Co-operative breeding in the anteating chat. *Ostrich*, **57**, 188–9.

Ebert, P. D. & Hyde, J. S. (1976). Selection for agonistic behavior in wild female *Mus musculus*. *Behavioral Genetics*, **6**, 291–304.

Eckhardt, R. C. (1976). Polygyny in the western wood pewee. *Condor*, **78**, 561–2.

Eisenberg, J. F. (1962). Studies on the behavior of *Peromyscus maniculatus gambelli* and *Peromyscus californicus parasiticus*. *Behaviour*, **19**, 177–207.

(1966). The social organization of mammals. In *Handbuch der Zoologie*. Berlin: Walter de Gruyter & Co.

(1968). Biology of promiscuous Rodentia. *Behavior Patterns*, **2**, 451–95.

(1981). *The Mammalian Radiations*. Chicago: University of Chicago Press.

Ekman, J. & Hake, M. (1988). Avian flocking reduces starvation risk: an experimental demonstration. *Behavioral Ecology and Sociobiology*, **22**, 91–4.

Elgar, M. A. (1986). The establishment of foraging flocks in house sparrows: risk of predation and daily temperature. *Behavioural Ecology and Sociobiology*, **19**, 433–8.

Elliott, P. F. (1980). Evolution of promiscuity in the brown-headed cowbird. *Condor*, **82**, 138–41.

Emlen, J. M. (1978). Territoriality: a fitness set-adaptive function approach. *American Naturalist*, **112**, 234–41.

Emlen, J. T., Jr. (1952). Flocking behavior in birds. *Auk*, **69**, 160–70.

Emlen, S. T. & Oring, L. W. (1977). Ecology, sexual selection and the evolution of mating systems. *Science*, **197**, 215–23.

204   *References*

Enders, R. K. (1945). Induced changes in the breeding habits of foxes. *Sociometry*, **8**, 53–5.

Erickson, J. G. (1967). Social hierarchy, territoriality, and stress reactions in sunfish. *Physiological Zoology*, **40**, 40–8.

Erlinge, S. (1967). Home range of the otter *Lutra lutra* L. in southern Sweden. *Oikos*, **18**, 186–209.

(1968). Territoriality of the otter *Lutra lutra* L. *Oikos*, **19**, 81–98.

Erlinge, S. & Sandell, M. (1986). Seasonal changes in the social organization of male stoats, *Mustela erminea*: an effect of shifts between two decisive resources. *Oikos*, **47**, 57–62.

Escherick, P. C. (1981). Social biology of the bushy-tailed woodrat, *Neotoma cinerea*. *University of California Publications in Zoology*, **110**.

Estes, R. D. (1966). Behaviour and life history of the wildebeest (*Connochaetes taurinus* Burchell). *Nature*, **212**, 999–1000.

Ettinger, A. E. & King, J. R. (1981). Consumption of green wheat enhances photostimulated ovarian growth in white-crowned sparrows. *Auk*, **98**, 832–4.

Evans, L. T. (1951). Field study of the social behavior of the black lizard, *Ctenosaura pectinata*. *American Museum Novitates*, 1495, 1–26.

(1953). Tail display in an iguanid lizard, *Liocephalus carinatus coryi*. *Copeia*, 1953, 50–4.

Faaborg, J. (1986). Reproductive success and survivorship of the Galapagos hawk *Buteo galapagoensis*: potential costs and benefits of cooperative polyandry. *Ibis*, **128**, 337–47.

Fabricius, E. & Boyd, H. (1985). A case of bigamy in the Canada goose. *Wildfowl*, **36**, 29–34.

Fabricius, E. & Gustafson, K.-J. (1953). Further aquarium observations on the spawning behaviour of the char, *Salmo alpinus* L. *Reports of the Institute of Freshwater Research, Drottningholm*, **35**, 58–104.

Ferguson, J. W. H., Nel, J. A. J. & deWet, M. J. (1983). Social organization and movement patterns of black-backed jackals *Canis mesomelas* in South Africa. *Journal of Zoology, London*, **199**, 487–502.

Ferron, J. & Ouellet, J. P. (1990). Temporal and intersexual variations in the use of space with regard to social organization in the woodchuck (*Marmota monax*). *Canadian Journal of Zoology*. (In press).

Fisler, G. F. (1965). Adaptation and speciation in harvest mice of the marshes of San Franciso Bay. *University of California Publications in Zoology*, **77**.

Fitch, M. A. & Shugart, G. W. (1983). Comparative biology and behavior of monogamous pairs and one male–two female trios of herring gulls. *Behavioral Ecology and Sociobiology*, **14**, 1–7.

Flinn, M. V. & Low, B. S. (1986). Resource distribution, social competition, and mating patterns in human societies. In *Ecological Aspects of Social Evolution*, ed. D. I. Rubenstein & R. W. Wrangham, pp. 217–43. Princeton, NJ: Princeton University Press.

Fraga, R. M. (1972). Cooperative breeding and a case of successive polyandry in the baywinged cowbird. *Auk*, **89**, 447–9.

(1979). Helpers at the nest in passerines from Buenos Aires Province, Argentina. *Auk*, **96**, 606–8.

Frame, G. & Frame, L. (1981). *Swift and Enduring*. New York: E. P. Dutton.

Francis, W. J. (1965). Double broods in California quail. *Condor*, **67**, 541–2.

Frank, F. (1957). The causality of microtine cycles in Germany. *Journal of Wildlife Management*, **21**, 113–21.

Frankel, O. H. & Soule, M. E. (1981). *Conservation and Evolution*. Cambridge: Cambridge University Press.

Franklin, W. L. (1983). Contrasting socioecologies of South America's wild camelids: the vicuna and the guanaco. *Advances in the Study of Mammalian Behavior*, **7**, 573–629.

Frankova, S. (1973). Effects of protein-calorie malnutrition on the development of social behaviour in the rat. *Developmental Psychobiology*, **15**, 21.

Freed, L. A. (1986a). Territory takeover and sexually selected infanticide in tropical house wrens. *Behavioral Ecology and sociobiology*, **19**, 197–206.

(1986b). Usurpatory and opportunistic bigamy in tropical house wrens. *Animal Behavior*, **34**, 1894–6.

Freeland, W. J. (1976). Pathogens and the evolution of primate sociality. *Biotropica*, **8**, 12–24.

(1977). Blood-sucking flies and primate polyspecific associations. *Nature*, **269**, 801–2.

(1979). Primate social groups as biological islands. *Ecology*, **60**, 719–28.

(1980). Mangabey (*Cercopithecus albigen*) movement patterns in relation to food availability and fecal contamination. *Ecology*, **61**, 1297–303.

(1981a). Functional aspects of primate grooming. *Ohio Academy of Sciences*, **81**, 173–7.

(1981b). Parasitism and behavioral dominance among male mice. *Science*, **213**, 416–2.

(1983). Parasites and the coexistence of animal host species. *American Naturalist*, **121**, 223–36.

Fricke, H. W. (1977). Community structure, social organization and ecological requirements of coral reef fish (Pomacentridae). *Holgander wiss. Meeresunters*, **30**, 412–26.

(1980). Mating systems, maternal and biparental care in triggerfish (*Balistidae*). *Zeitschrift für Tierpsychologie*, **53**, 105–22.

Friedman, M. H. & Friedman, G. S. (1939). Gonadotrophic extracts from green leaves. *American Journal of Physiology*, **124**, 486–90.

Frith, H. J. & Davies, S. J. J. F. (1961). Ecology of the magpie goose, *Anseranas semipalmata* Latham (Anatidae). *C.S.I.R.O. Wildlife Research*, 1961, 91–141.

Fry, C. H. (1972). The social organisation of bee-eaters (Meropidae) and co-operative breeding in hot-climate birds. *Ibis*, **114**, 1–14.

Fulk, K. R., Logan, C. A. & Hyatt, L. E. (1987). Polyandry in a female northern mockingbird. *Wilson Bulletin*, **99**, 286–8.

Galef, B. G. Jr. (1988). Imitation in animals: history, definition, and interpretation of data from the psychological laboratory. In *Social Learning, Psycho-*

logical and Biological Perspectives, ed. T. R. Zentall & B. G. Galef, Jr., pp. 3–28. Hillsdale, NJ: Lawrence Erlbaum Assoc.

Galef, B. G. Jr. & Clark, M. M. (1971). Social factors in the poison avoidance and feeding behavior of wild and domesticated rat pups. *Journal of Comparative Physiology and Psychology*, **75**, 341–57.

Ganslosser, U. (1980). An annotated bibliography of social behaviour in kangaroos (Macropodidae). *Sonderdruck aus Saugetierkundliche Mitteilungen*, **40**, 138–48.

Garcia, J. F. & Koelling, R. A. (1966). Relation of cue to consequence in avoidance learning. *Psychonomic Science*, **4**, 123–4.

Garnett, S. T. (1978). The behaviour patterns of the dusky moorhen, *Gallinula tenebrosa* Gould (Aves: Rallidae). *Australian Wildlife Research*, **5**, 363–84.

(1980). The social organization of the dusky moorhen, *Gallinula tenebrosa* Gould (Aves: Rallidae). *Australian Wildlife Research*, **7**, 103–12.

Gates, S. (1979). A study of the home ranges of free-ranging Exmoor ponies. *Mammal Review*, **9**, 3–18.

Gauthier, G. (1986). Experimentally-induced polygyny in buffleheads: evidence for a mixed reproductive strategy? *Animal Behaviour*, **34**, 300–2.

Geist, V. (1971). *Mountain Sheep*. Chicago: University of Chicago Press.

(1981). Behavior: adaptive strategies in mule deer. In *Mule and Black-tailed Deer of North America*, ed. O. C. Walmo, pp. 157–224. Lincoln: University of Nebraska Press.

Getz, L. L., Hofmann, J. E. & Carter, C. S. (1987). Mating system and population fluctuations of the prairie vole, *Microtus ochrogaster*. *American Zoologist*, **27**, 909–20.

Gibbons, D. W. (1986). Brood parasitism and cooperative nesting in the moorhen, *Gallinula chloropus*. *Behavioural Ecology and Sociobiology*, **19**, 221–32.

Gibson, R. M. & Bradbury, J. W. (1987). Lek organization in sage grouse: variations on a territorial theme. *Auk*, **104**, 77–84.

Gilbert, D. L. (1978). Evolution and taxonomy. In *Big Game of North America*, ed. J. L. Schmidt & D. L. Gilbert, pp. 1–9. Harrisburg, PA: Stackpole Books.

Gill, F. B. & Wolf, L. L. (1975). Economics of feeding territoriality in the golden-winged sunbird. *Ecology*, **56**, 333–45.

Ginetz, R. M. & Larkin, P. A. (1976). Factors affecting rainbow trout (*Salmo gairdneri*) predation on migrant fry of sockeye salmon (*Oncorhynchus nerka*). *Journal of Fisheries Research Board of Canada*, **33**, 19–24.

Gittleman, J. L. (1989). Carnivore group living: comparative trends. In *Carnivore Behavior, Ecology and Evolution*, ed. J. L. Gittleman, pp. 183–207. Ithaca, NY: Cornell University Press.

Glazener, W. C. (1967). Management of the Rio Grande turkey. In *The Wild Turkey and its Management*, ed. O. H. Hewitt, pp. 453–92. Washington, DC: The Wildlife Society.

Goeden, G. B. (1978). A monograph of the coral trout *Plectropomus leopardus* (Lacepede). *Queensland Fisheries Service Research Bulletin*, **1**, 1–42.

Goldizen, A. W. (1987). Facultative polyandry and the role of infant-carrying in wild saddle-back tamarins (*Saguinus fuscicollis*). *Behavioural Ecology and Sociobiology*, **20**, 99–109.

(1988). Tamarin and marmoset mating systems: unusual flexibility. *Trends in Ecology and Evolution*, **3**, 36–40.

Gosling, L. M. (1986). The evolution of the mating strategies in male antelopes. In *Ecological Aspects of Social Evolution*, ed. D. I. Rubenstein & R. W. Wrangham, pp. 244–81. Princeton, NJ: Princeton University Press.

(1987). Scent marking in an antelope lek territory. *Animal Behaviour*, **35**, 620–2.

Gosling, L. M. (1990). *Applied Animal Behavior*. (In press.)

Gosling, L. M., Petrie, M. & Rainy, M. E. (1987). Lekking in topi: a high cost, specialist strategy. *Animal Behaviour*, **35**, 616–18.

Gould, S. J. & Lewontin, R. C. (1979). The spandrels of San Marco and the Panglossian paradigm: a critique of the adaptationist programme. *Proceedings of the Royal Society of London*, **205B**, 581–98.

Gowaty, P. A. (1981). An extension of the Orians-Verner-Willson model to account for mating systems besides polygyny. *American Naturalist*, **118**, 851–9.

(1983). Male parental care and apparent monogamy among eastern bluebirds *Sialia sialis*. *American Naturalist*, **121**, 149–57.

Gowaty, P. A. & Karlin, A. A. (1984). Multiple maternity and paternity in single broods of apparently monogamous eastern bluebirds (*Sialia sialis*). *Behavioral Ecology and Sociobiology*, **15**, 91–5.

Graul, W. D. (1973). Adaptive aspects of the mountain plover social system. *Living Bird*, **12**, 69–94.

Green, P. T. (1982). Bigamy in the rook *Corvus frugilegus*. *Ibis*, **124**, 193–6.

Greenberg, B. (1947). Some relations between territory, social hierarchy, and leadership in the green sunfish (*Lepomis cyanellus*). *Physiological Zoology*, **20**, 267–99.

Greene, E. (1987). Individuals in an osprey colony discriminate between high and low quality information. *Nature*, **329**, 239–41.

Greeves, N. (1926). Nine eggs of sparrow hawk in same nest. *British Birds*, **20**, 77.

Griffin, D. R. (1984). *Animal Thinking*. Cambridge, MA: Harvard University Press.

Grimes, L. G. (1973). The breeding of Heuglin's masked weaver and its nesting association with the red weaver ant. *Ostrich*, **44**, 170–5.

Gross, M. R. (1982). Sneakers, satellites and parentals: polymorphic mating strategies in North American sunfishes. *Zeitschrift für Tierpsychologie*, **60**, 1–26.

(1983). Sunfish, salmon, and the evolution of alternative reproductive strategies and tactics in fishes. In *Fish Reproduction: Strategies and Tactics*, ed. R. J. Wootton & G. Potts, pp. 55–75. New York: Academic Press.

Gross, M. R. & Charnov, E. L. (1980). Alternative male life histories in bluegill sunfish. *Proceedings of the National Academy of Sciences*, **77**, 6937–40.

Hall, K. R. L. & Goswell, M. J. (1964). Aspects of social learning in captive patas monkeys. *Primates*, **5**, 59–70.

Hamerstrom, F., Hamerstrom, F. N. & Burke, C. J. (1985). Effect of voles on mating systems in a central Wisconsin population of harriers. *Wilson Bulletin*, **97**, 332–46.

Hamilton, W. D. (1964a). The genetical evolution of social behaviour. I. *Journal of Theoretical Biology*, **7**, 1–16.

(1964b). The genetical evolution of social behaviour. II. *Journal of Theoretical Biology*, **7**, 17–32.

(1971). Geometry for the selfish herd. *Journal of Theoretical Biology*, **31**, 295–311.

Hamilton, W. D. & Zuk, M. (1984). Heritable true fitness and bright birds: a role for parasites? *Science*, **218**, 384–7.

Hamilton, W. J. III & Watt, K. E. F. (1970). Refuging. *Annual Review of Ecology and Systematics*, **1**, 263–86.

Hann, H. W. (1940). Polyandry in the oven-bird. *Wilson Bulletin*, **52**, 69–72.

(1983). Spacing and breeding density of willow ptarmigan in response to an experimental alteration of sex ratio. *Journal of Animal Ecology*, **52**, 807–20.

Hannon, S. J. (1983). Spacing and breeding density of willow ptarmigan in response to an experimental alteration of sex ratio. *Journal of Animal Ecology*, **52**, 807–20.

(1984). Factors limiting polygyny in the willow ptarmigan. *Animal Behaviour*, **32**, 153–61.

Hannon, S. J., Mumme, R. L., Koenig, W. D., Spon, S. & Pitelka, F. A. (1987). Poor acorn crop, dominance, and decline in numbers of acorn woodpeckers. *Journal of Animal Ecology*, **56**, 197–207.

Harcourt, A. H., Fossey, D., Stewart, K. J. & Watts, D. P. (1980). Reproduction in wild gorillas and some comparisons with chimpanzees. *Journal of Reproduction and Fertility*, Supplement, **28**, 59–70.

Hardin, J. W., Silvy, N. J. & Klimstra, W. D. (1976). Group size and composition of the Florida key deer. *Journal of Wildlife Management*, **40**, 454–63.

Harper, D. (1986). Bigamy by treecreepers. *British Birds*, **79**, 250.

Harper, D. G. C. (1985). Brood division in robins. *Animal Behavior*, **33**, 466–80.

Harris, M. P. (1982). Promiscuity in the shag as shown by time-lapse photography. *Bird Study*, **29**, 149–54.

Hart, B. L. (1988). Biological basis of the behavior of sick animals. *Neuroscience and Biobehavioral Reviews*, **12**, 123–37.

Harvey, P. H., Stenning, M. J. & Campbell, B. (1985). Individual variation in seasonal breeding success of pied flycatchers (*Ficedula hypolecua*). *Journal of Animal Ecology*, **54**, 391–8.

Hatch, J. J. (1975). Piracy by laughing gulls *Larus atricilla*: an example of the selfish group. *Ibis*, **117**, 357–65.

Hay, D. A. (1985). *Essentials of Behaviour Genetics*. Melbourne: Blackwell.

Hennessy, D. F. (1986). On the deadly risk of predator harassment. *Ethology*, **72**, 72–4.

Hilden, O. (1975). Breeding system of Temminck's stint *Calidris temminckii*. *Ornis Fennica.*, **52**, 117–46.

Hill, J. (1978). The origin of sociocultural evolution. *Journal of Social Biology Structure*, **1**, 377–86.

Hinde, R. A. (1976). Interactions, relationships and social structure. *Man*, **11**, 1–17.

(1983). A conceptual framework. In *Primate Social Relationships*, ed. R. A. Hinde, pp. 1–7. Oxford: Blackwell Scientific Publications.

Hirth, D. H. (1977). Social behavior of white-tailed deer in relation to habitat. *Wildlife Monographs*, **53**, 1–55.

Hoff, J. G. (1984). Observations on male ruffed grouse, *Bonasa umbellus*, accompanying brood. *Canadian Field-naturalist*, **98**, 49–50.

Hoffmann, R. (1983). Social organization patterns of several feral horse and feral ass populations in central Australia. *Zeitschrift für Saeugetierkunde*, **48**, 124–6.

Hogg, J. T. (1988). Copulatory tactics in relation to sperm competition in Rocky Mountain bighorn sheep. *Behavioral Ecology and Sociobiology*, **22**, 49–59.

Houston, A. I. & Davies, N. B. (1985). The evolution of cooperation and life history in the dunnock, *Prunella modularis*. In *Behavioural Ecology: Ecological Consequences of Adaptive Behaviour*, ed. R. M. Sibly & R. H. Smith, pp. 471–87. Oxford: Blackwell Scientific Publications.

Howard, H. E. (1920). *Territory in Bird Life*. London: John Murray.

Howard, R. D. (1978). The evolution of mating strategies in bullfrogs, *Rana catesbiana*. *Evolution*, **32**, 850–71.

Howard, W. E. (1950). Relation between low temperature and available food to survival of small rodents. *Journal of Mammalogy*, **32**, 300–12.

Howe, H. F. (1979). Evolutionary aspects of parental care in the common grackle, *Quiscalus quiscula* L. *Evolution*, **33**, 41–51.

Howe, R. W. & Noske, R. A. (1979). Cooperative feeding of fledglings by crested shrike-tits. *Emu*, **80**, 40.

Hunt, G. L. Jr. & Hunt, M. W. (1977). Female-female pairing in western gulls (*Larus occidentalis*) in southern California. *Science*, **196**, 1466–7.

Hunter, L. A. (1987a). Acquisition of territories by floaters in cooperatively breeding purple gallinules. *Animal Behaviour*, **35**, 402–10.

(1987b). Cooperative breeding in purple gallinules: the role of helpers in feeding chicks. *Behavioral Ecology and Sociobiology*, **20**, 171–7.

Hurley, T. A. & Robertson, R. J. (1984). Aggressive and territorial behaviour in female red-winged blackbirds. *Canadian Journal of Zoology*, **62**, 148–53.

Hurst, J. L. (1987). Behavioural variation in wild house mice *Mus domesticus rutty*: a quantitative assessment of female social organization. *Animal Behavior*, **35**, 1846–57.

Itani, J. & Nishimura, A. (1973). The study of infrahuman culture in Japan: a review. *Symposium of the 4th International Congress on Primatology*, **1**, 26–50.

Ivanitzky, V. V. (1978). Ecological and behavioural prerequisites of polygyny in the isabelline chat *Oenanthe isabellina* (Aves, Turdidae). *Zoologicheskii Zhurnal*, **57**, 1555–65.

Izumi, T. (1973). Social behaviour of the Norway rat (*R. norvegicus*) in their natural habitat (especially on their group types). *Japanese Journal of Ecology*, **23**, 55–64.

James, P. C. & Oliphant, L. W. (1986). Extra birds and helpers at the nests of Richardson's merlin. *Condor*, **88**, 533–4.

Jarman, M. V. (1979). Impala social behavior. Territory, hierarchy, mating and the uses of space. *Advances in Ethology*, **21**.

Jarman, P. J. (1974). The social organization of antelope in relation to their ecology. *Behaviour*, **48**, 215–66.

Jarman, P. J. & Jarman, M. V. (1974). Impala behaviour and its relevance to management. In *The Behaviour of Ungulates and its Relation to Management*, ed. V. Geist & F. Walther, pp. 871–81. Morges, Switzerland: IUCN.

Jenkins, T. M. Jr. (1969). Social structure, position choice and microdistribution of two trout species (*Salmo trutta* and *Salmo gairdneri*) resident in mountain streams. *Animal Behaviour Monographs*, **2**, 57–123.

(1971). Role of social behavior in dispersal of introduced rainbow trout (*Salmo gairdneri*). *Journal of Fisheries Research Board of Canada*, **28**, 1019–27.

Johns, D. W. & Armitage, K. B. (1979). Behavioral ecology of alpine yellow-bellied marmots. *Behavioural Ecology and Sociobiology*, **5**, 133–57.

Jourdain, F. C. R. (1926a). Polygamy in the sparrow hawk. *British Birds*, **19**, 180.

(1926b). Polygamy in the Accipitres. *British Birds*, **19**, 314.

Jouventin, P. & Cornet, A. (1980). The sociobiology of pinnipeds. *Advances in the Study of Behavior*, **11**, 121–41.

Jungius, H. (1971). The biology and behaviour of the reedbuck (*Redunca arundinum* Boddaert 1875) in the Kruger National Park. *Mammalia depicta*, **6**.

Kalas, J. A. (1986). Incubation schedules in different parental care systems in the dotterel *Charadrius morinelius*. *Ardea*, **74**, 185–90.

Kalleberg, H. (1958). Observations in a stream tank of territoriality and competition in juvenile salmon and trout (*Salmo salar* L. and *Salmo trutta* L.) *Reports of the Institute of Freshwater Research, Drottingholm*, **39**, 55–98.

Karstad, E. L. & Hudson R. J. (1986). Social organization and communication of riverine hippopotami in southwestern Kenya. *Mammalia*, **50**, 153–64.

Kattan, G. (1988). Food habits and social organization of acorn woodpeckers in Colombia. *Condor*, **90**, 100–6.

Kavanau, J. L. (1988). Presumptive relict reproductive behavior in small parrots. *Brain Behavioral Ecology*, **32**, 340–52.

Kawanabe, H. (1972). An evolutionary aspect of the territoriality of ayu-fish, *Plecoglossus altivelis*, with the social structure at the southern end of its distribution. *Japanese Journal of Ecology*, **22**, 141–9.

Keenleyside, M. H. A. (1985). Bigamy and mate choice in the biparental cichlid fish *Cichlasoma nigrofasciatum*. *Behavioural Ecology and Sociobiology*, **17**, 285–90.

Keenleyside, M. H. A. & Yamamoto, F. T. (1962). Territorial behaviour of juvenile Atlantic salmon (*salmo salar* L.). *Behaviour*, **19**, 139–69.

Kendeigh, S. C. (1941). Territorial and mating behavior of the house wren. *Illinois Biological Monographys*, **18**, 1–120.

Kenward, R. E. (1978). Hawks and doves: factors affecting success and selection in goshawk attacks on wood pigeons. *Journal of Animal Ecology*, **47**, 449–60.

Kilham, L. (1984). Intra- and extrapair copulatory behavior of American crows. *Wilson Bulletin*, **96**, 716–7.

Kiltie, R. A. & Fitzpatrick, J. W. (1984). Reproduction and social organization of the black-capped donacobius in southeastern Peru. *Auk*, **101**, 804–11.

Kinsey, K. P. (1971). Social organization in a laboratory colony of wood rats *Neotoma fuscipes*. In *Behaviour and Environment: The Use of Space by Animals and Men*, ed. A. H. Esser, pp. 40-5. New York: Plenum Press.

(1977). Agonistic behavior and social organization in a reproductive population of allegheny woodrats, *Neotoma floridana magister*. *Journal of Mammalogy*, **58**, 417–19.

Kitchen, D. W. (1974). Social behavior and ecology of the pronghorn. *Wildlife Monographs*, **38**.

Kleiman, D. G. (1977). Monogamy in mammals. *Quarterly Review of Biology*, **52**, 39–69.

Klein, L. L. & Klein, D. B. (1977). Feeding behaviour of the Colombian spider monkey. In *Primate Ecology*, ed. T. H. Clutton-Brock, pp. 153–81. New York: Academic Press.

Knowles, E. H. M. (1938). Polygamy in the western lark sparrow. *Auk*, **55**, 675–6.

Kodric-Brown, A. & Brown, J. H. (1978). Influence of economics, interspecific competition and sexual dimorphism on territoriality of migrant rufous hummingbirds. *Ecology*, **59**, 285–96.

Koenig, W. D., Munne, R. L. & Pitelka, F. A. (1984). The breeding system of the acorn woodpecker in central coastal California. *Zeitschrift für Tierpsychologie*, **65**, 289–308.

Koford, R. R., Bowen, B. S. & Vehrencamp, S. L. (1986). Habitat saturation in groove-billed anis (*Crotophaga sulcirostris*). *American Naturalist*, **127**, 317–37.

Kolb, H. H. (1986). Some observations on the home ranges of vixens (*Vulpes vulpes*) in the suburbs of Edinburgh. *Journal of Zoology*, **210**, 636–9.

Komeda, S., Yamagishi, S. & Fujioka, M. (1987). Cooperative breeding in azurewinged magpies, *Cyanopica cyana*, living in a region of heavy snowfall. *Condor*, **89**, 835–41.

Kossack, C. W. (1950). Breeding habits of Canada geese under refuge conditions. *American Midland Naturalist*, **43**, 627–49.

Kovacs, K. M. & Ryder, J. P. (1983). Reproductive performance of female-female pairs and polygynous trios of ring-billed gulls. *Auk*, **100**, 658–69.

Krebs, J. R. (1974). Colonial nesting and social feeding as strategies for exploiting food resources in the great blue heron (*Ardea herodias*). *Behaviour*, **51**, 99–134.

Krebs, J. R. & Davies, N. B. (1987). *An Introduction to Behavioural Ecology*. Sunderland, MA: Sinauer Associates, Inc.

Krekorian, C. O. (1978). Alloparental care in the purple gallinule. *Condor*, **80**, 382–90.

Kroodsma, D. E. & Canady, R. A. (1985). Differences in repertoire size, singing behavior, and associated neuroanatomy among marsh wren populations have a genetic basis. *Auk*, **102**, 439–46.

Kruuk, H. (1972). *The Spotted Hyena*. Chicago: University of Chicago Press.

(1975). Functional aspects of social hunting by carnivores. In *Function and Evolution in Behavior*, ed. G. Baerends, C. Beer, & A. Manning. Oxford: Clarendon Press.

(1976). Feeding and social behavior of the striped hyaena (*Hyaena vulgaris* Desmarest). *East African Wildlife Journal*, **14**, 91–111.

(1986). The case of the clannish bader. *Natural History*, **95**, 50–7.

Kruuk, H. & Hewson, R. (1978). Spacing and foraging of otters (*Lutra lutra*) in a marine habitat. *Journal of Zoology, London*, **185**, 205–12.

Kruuk, H. & Parish, T. (1982). Factors affecting population density, group size and territory size of the European badger, *Meles meleo*. *Journal of Zoology, London*, **196**, 31–9.

(1987). Changes in the size of groups and ranges of the European badger (*Meles meles* L.) in an area in Scotland. *Journal of Animal Ecology*, **56**, 351–64.

Kushlan, J. A. (1973). Promiscuous mating behavior in the white ibis. *Wilson Bulletin*, **85**, 331–2.

Lack, D. (1968). *Ecological Adaptations for Breeding in Birds*. London: Methuen & Co. Ltd.

LaGrenade, M-C. & Mousseau, P. (1983). Female-female pairs and polygynous associations in a Quebec ring-billed gull colony. *Auk*, 100, 210–12.

Laine, H. (1981). Male participation in incubation and brooding in the blue jay. *Auk*, **98**, 622–3.

Lamprecht, J. (1987). Female reproductive strategies in bar- headed geese (*Anser indicus*): why are geese monogamous? *Behavioral Ecology and Sociobiology*, **21**, 297–305.

Lamprecht, J. & Buhrow, H. (1987). Harem polgyny in bar-headed geese. *Ardea*, **75**, 285–92.

Lane, R. (1978). Co-operative breeding in the Australian little grebe. *Sunbird*, **9**, 2.

Laskey, A. R. (1947). Evidence of polyandry at a bluebird nest. *Auk*, **64**, 314–15.

Lawn, M. R. (1978). Bigamous willow warbler. *British Birds*, **71**, 592–3.

Layne, J. N. (1954). The biology of the red squirrel, *Tamiasciurus hudsonicus loquax* (Bangs), in central New York. *Ecological Monographs*, **24**, 227–67.

Lazarus, T. (1979). The early warning function of flocking in birds: an experimental study with captive guides. *Animal Behavior*, **27**, 855–65.

Le Boeuf, B. J. (1986). Sexual strategies of seals and walruses. *New Scientist*, **16** January, 36–9.

Lederer, R. J. (1981). Facultative territoriality in Townsend's solitaire (*Myadestes townsendi*). *Southwestern Naturalist*, **25**, 461–7.

Lenington, S. (1980). Bi-parental care in killdeer: an adaptive hypothesis. *Wilson Bulletin*, **92**, 8–20.

Lennartz, M. R., Hooper, R. G. & Harlow, R. F. (1987). Sociality and cooperative breeding of red-cockaded woodpeckers, *Picoides borealis*. *Behavioural Ecology and Sociobiology*, **20**, 77–88.

Lent, P. C. (1969). A preliminary study of the Okavago lechwe *Kobus leche leche* (Gray). *East African Wildlife Journal*, **7**, 147–57.

Leopold, A. S. (1944). The nature of heritable wildness in turkeys. *Condor*, **46**, 133–97.

(1977). *The California Quail*. Berkeley: University of California Press.

Leopold, A. S., Ervin, M., Oh, J. & Browning, B. (1976). Phytoestrogens: adverse effects on reproduction in California quail. *Science*, **191**, 98–100.

Lessells, C. M. (1984). The mating system of Kentish plovers *Charadrius alexandrinus*. *Ibis*, **126**, 474–83.

Leuthold, W. (1966). Variations in territorial behavior of Uganda kob *Adentota kob thomasi* (Neumann 1896). *Behaviour*, **27**, 215–57.

(1977). African ungulates: a comparative review of their ethology and behavioural ecology. *Zoophysiology and Ecology*, vol. **8**.

Levesley, P. B. & Magurran, A. E. (1988). Population differences in the reaction of minnows to alarm substance. *Journal of Fish Biology*, **32**, 699–706.

Lewis, D. M. (1982). Cooperative breeding in a population of white-browed sparrow weavers *Plocepasser mahali*. *Ibis*, **124**, 511–22.

Lewis, R. A. (1985). Do blue grouse form leks? *Auk*, **102**, 180–4.

Lewontin, R. C. (1979). Sociobiology as an adaptationist program. *Behavioral Science*, **24**, 4–14.

Leyhausen, P. (1965). The communal organization of solitary mammals. *Symposia of the Zoological Society of London*, **14**, 249–63.

Ligon, J. D. & Ligon, S. H. (1988). Territory quality: key determinant of fitness in the group-living green woodhoopoe. In *The Ecology of Social Behavior*, ed. C. N. Slobodchikoff, pp. 229–53. San Diego: Academic Press, Inc.

Limberger, D. (1983). Pairs and harems in a cichlid fish, *Lamprologus brichardi*. *Zeitschrift für Tierpsychologie*, **62**, 115–44.

Lloyd, C. W. & Weisz, J. (1975). Hormones and aggression. In *Neural Bases of Violence and Aggression*, ed. W. S. Fields, & W. H. Sweet, pp. 92–127. W. H. Green.

Logan, C. A. & Rulli, M. (1981). Bigamy in a male mockingbird. *Auk*, **98**, 385–6.

Lombardo, M. P. (1986). Extrapair copulations in the tree swallow. *Wilson Bulletin*, **98**, 150–2.

Lott, D. F. (1979). Dominance relations and breeding rate in mature male American bison. *Zeitschrift für Tierpsychologie*, **49**, 418–32.

(1984). Intraspecific variation in the social systems of wild vertebrates. *Behaviour*, **88**, 266–325.

Lott, D. F. & Minta, S. C. (1983). Random individual association and social group instability in American bison (*Bison bison*). *Zeitschrift für Tierpsychologie*, **61**, 153–72.

MacDonald, D. W. (1978). Observations on the behaviour and ecology of the striped hyaena, *Hyaena hyaena*, in Israel. *Israel Journal of Zoology*, **27**, 189–98.

(1979). 'Helpers' in fox society. *Nature*, **282**, 69–71.

(1980). Social factors affecting reproduction amongst red foxes, *Vulpes vulpes*. *Biogeographica*, **18**, 123–75.

(1981). Resource dispersion and the social organization of the red fox (*Vulpes vulpes*). *Worldwide Furbearers Conference Proceedings*, **2**, 918–49.

(1983). The ecology of carnivore social behavior. *Nature*, **301**, 379–84.

MacDonald, D. W., Apps, P. J., Carr, G. M. & Kerby, G. (1987). *Social Dynamics, Nursing Coalitions, and Infanticide among Farm Cats*, Felis catus. Berlin: Paul Parey Scientific Publishers.

MacDonald, S. M. & Mason, C. F. (1980). Observations on the marking behaviour of a coastal population of otters. *Acta Theriologica*, **25**, 245–53.

MacRoberts, M. H. & MacRoberts, B. R. (1976). Social organization and behavior of the acorn woodpecker in central coastal California. *Ornithological Monographs*, **21**, 1–115.

Mader, W. J. (1975a). Biolgoy of the Harris' hawk in southern Arizona. *Living Bird*, **14**, 59–84.

(1975b). Extra adults at Harris' hawk nests. *Condor*, **77**, 482–5.

(1977). Harris' hawks lay three clutches of eggs in one year. *Auk*, **94**, 370–1.

(1979). Breeding behavior of a polyandrous trio of Harris' hawks in southern Arizona. *Auk*, **96**, 776–8.

Mainardi, D. (1980). Tradition and the social transmission of behavior in animals. In *Sociobiology: Beyond Nature/Nurture?* ed. G. W. Barlow & J. Silverberg, pp. 227–55. Boulder, CO: Westview Press, Inc.

Malcolm, J. R. (1986). Socio-ecology of bat-eared foxes (*Otocyon megalotis*). *Journal of Zoology*, **208**, 457–67.

Manzur, M. I. & Fuentes, E. R. (1979). Polygyny and agonistic behavior in the tree-dwelling lizard *Liolaemus tenuis* (Iguanidae). *Behavioural Ecology and Sociobiology*, **6**, 23–8.

Marchinton, R. L. & Atkeson, T. D. (1985). Plasticity of soci-spatial behaviour of white-tailed deer and the concept of facultative territoriality. In *Biology of Deer Production*, ed. P. F. Fennessy & K. R. Drew, pp. 375–7. Wellington: Royal Society of New Zealand.

Marks, J., Doremus, J. & Marks, V. S. (1987). Polygyny in the northern saw-whet owl. Presented at the 57th Annual Meeting of the Cooper Ornithological Society, June 21–26, 1987, Snowbird, Utah.

Marti, C. D. (1987). Polygyny in the common barn-owl. Presented at the 57th Annual Meeting of the Cooper Ornithological Society, June 21–26, 1987, Snowbird, Utah.

Martin, K. (1984). Reproductive defence priorities of male willow ptarmigan (*Lagopus lagopus*): enhancing mate survival or extending paternity options? *Behavioural Ecology and Sociobiology*, **16**, 57–63.

(1989). Pairing and adoption of offspring by replacement male willow ptarmigan: behavior, costs and consequences. *Animal Behavior*, **37**, 569–78.

Martin, K. & Hannon, S. J. (1987). Natal philopatry and recruitment of willow ptarmigan in north central and northwestern Canada. *Oecologia*, **71**, 518–24.

Martin, P. & Bateson, P. (1987). *Measuring Behaviour*. Cambridge: Cambridge University Press.

Martin, S. G. (1974). Adaptations for polygynous breeding in the bobolink, *Dolichonyx oryzivorus*. *American Zoologist*, **14**, 109–19.

Mason, W. (1979). Ontogeny of social behavior. *Handbook of Behavioral Neurobiology*, **3**, 1–28.

Mason, W. A. (1984). Animal learning: experience, life modes and cognitive style. *Verhandlingen, Deutscher Zoologie Gesellschaft*, **77**, 45–56.

(1986). Behavior implies cognition. In *Integrating Scientific Disciplines*, ed. W. Bechtel, pp. 297–307. Dordrecht: Martinus Nijhoff.

Matthysen, E. (1986). Some observations on sex-specific territoriality in the nuthatch. *Ardea*, **74**, 177–83.

Maublanc, M.-L., Bideau, E. & Vincent, J.-P. (1987). Flexibilité de l'organisation sociale du chevreuil en fonction des carasteristiques de l'environnement. *Review of Ecology*, **42**, 109–33.

Maxson, S. J. & Oring, L. W. (1980). Breeding season time and energy budgets of the polyandrous spotted sandpiper. *Behaviour*, **74**, 200–63.

May, R. (1988). Conservation and disease. *Conservation Biology*, **2**, 28–30.

Maynard Smith, J. (1974). The theory of games and the resolution of animal conflict. *Journal of Theoretical Biology*, **47**, 209–21.

(1976). Evolution and the theory of games. *American Scientist*, **64**, 41–5.

(1978). *The Evolution of Sex*. Cambridge: Cambridge University Press.

(1982). *Evolution and the Theory of Games*. Cambridge: Cambridge University Press.

Mays, N. A., Vleck, C. M., Dawson, J. W. & Mannan, R. W. (1989). Correlations of steroid hormones with reproductive behavior in breeders and helpers in the cooperatively breeding Harris' hawk. Presented at the 107th meeting of the American Ornithologists; Union, Pittsburgh, Pennsylvania. 7–10 August 1989.

McBride, G., Parer, I. P. & Foenander, F. (1969). The social organization and behaviour of the feral domestic fowl. *Animal Behaviour Monographs*, **2**, 127–81.

McCartan, L. & Simmons, K. E. L. (1956). Territory in the great crested grebe *Podiceps cristatus* re-examined. *Ibis*, **98**, 370–8.

McKinney, F. (1986). Ecological factors influencing the social systems of migratory dabbling ducks. In *Ecological Aspects of Social Evolution*, ed. D. I. Rubenstein & R. W. Wrangham, pp. 153–71. Princeton, NJ: Princeton University Press.

McKinney, F., Siegfried, W. R., Ball, I. J. & Frost, P. G. (1978). Behavioral specializations for river life in the African black duck *Anas sparse eyton*. *Zeitschrift für Tierpsychologie*, **48**, 349–400.

M'Closkey, R. T. Baia, K. A. & Russell, R. W. (1987). Tree lizard (*Urosaurus ornatus*) territories: experimental perturbation of the ratio. *Ecology*, **68**, 2059–62.

McMillan, I. I. (1964). Annual population changes in California quail. *Journal of Wildlife Management*, **28**, 702–11.

McNair, D. B. (1985). An auxiliary with a mated pair and food- caching behavior in the fish crow. *Wilson Bulletin*, **97**, 123–5.

Mech, L. D. (1970). *The Wolf: the Ecology and Behavior of an Endangered Species*. Garden City, NY: Natural History Press.

Mendelsohn, J. (1988). Communal roosting and feeding conditions in blackshouldered kites. *Ostrich*, **59**, 73–5.

Michener, H. (1925). Polygamy practiced by the house finch. *Condor*, **27**, 116.

Mihok, S. (1979). Behavioural structure and demography of subarctic *Clethrionomys gapperi* and *Peromyscus maniculatus*. *Canadian Journal of Zoology*, **57**, 1520–35.

Miller, D. R. (1979). Wolf-caribou-human interactions on the taiga of northcentral Canada during winter. In *The Behavior and Ecology of Wolves*, ed. E. Klinghammer, pp. 93–116. New York: Garland STPM Press.

Miller, F. L. (1974). Four types of territoriality observed in a herd of black-tailed deer. In *The Behaviour of Ungulates and its Relation to Management*, ed. V. Geist & F. Walther, pp. 644–60. Morges, Switzerland: IUCN.

Miller, G. R. & Watson, A. (1978). Territories and the food plant of individual red grouse. *Journal of Animal Ecology*, **47**, 293–305.

Miller, R. (1981). Male aggression, dominance and breeding behavior in Red Desert feral horses. *Zeitschrift für Tierpsychologie*, **57**, 340–51.

Mills, M. G. L. (1982). The mating system of the brown hyaena, *Hyaena brunnea* in the southern Kalahari. *Behavioral Ecology and Sociobiology*, **10**, 131–6.

Mitchell, G. J. (1971). Measurements, weights and carcass yields of pronghorns in Alberta. *Journal of Wildlife Management*, **35**, 76–85.

Mochek, A. D. & Valdes-Munoz, E. (1983). Influencia del relieve del fondo sobre la conducta gregaria de los peces. *Ciencias Biologicas*, **9**, 79–85.

Moehlman, P. D. (1979). Jackal helpers and pup survival. *Nature*, **277**, 382–3.
  (1986). Ecology of cooperation in canids. In *Ecological Aspects of Social Evolution*, ed. D. I. Rubenstein & R. W. Wrangham, pp. 64–86. Princeton, NJ: Princeton University Press.
  (1989). Intraspecific variation in canid social system. In *Carnivore Behavior, Ecology and Evolution*, ed. J. L. Gittleman, pp. 143–63. Ithaca: Cornell University Press.

Moller, A. P. (1983). Habitat selection and feeding activity in the magpie *Pica pica*. *Journal für Ornithologie*, **124**, 147–61.

Monaghan, P. & Metcalfe, N. B. (1985). Group foraging in wild brown hares: effects of resource distribution and social status. *Animal Behaviour*, **33**, 993–9.

Monfort-Brahm, N. (1975). Variations dans la structure sociale du topi, *Damaliscus korrigum* Ogilby, au Parc National de l'Akagera, Rwanda. *Zeitschrift für Tierpsychologie*, **39**, 332–64.

Montevecchi, W. A. (1979). Predator–prey interactions between ravens and kittiwakes. *Zeitschrift für Tierpsychologie*, **49**, 136–41.

Mousseau, T. A. & Collins, N. C. (1987). Polygyny and nest site abundance in the slimy sculpin (*Cottus cognatus*). *Canadian Journal of Zoology*, **65**, 2827–9.

Muldal, A. M., Moffatt, J. D. & Robertson, R. J. (1986). Parental care of nestlings by male red-winged blackbirds. *Behavioral Ecology and Sociobiology*, **19**, 105–14.

Mumford, R. E. (1964). The breeding biology of the Acadian flycatcher. *Miscellaneous Publications, Museum of Zoology, Universtiy of Michigan*, **125**, 1–50.

Mumme, R. L., Koenig, W. D. & Pitelka, F. A. (1988). Costs and benefits of joint nesting in the acorn woodpecker. *American Naturalist*, **131**, 654–77.

Munro, A. D. & Singh, I. (1987). Diurnal changes in the territorial behaviour of the tilapia *Oreochromis mossambicus* (Peters). *Journal of Fish Biology*, **30**, 459–64.

Munro, J. & Bedard, J. (1977). Gull predation and creching behaviour in the common eider. *Journal of Animal Ecology*, **46**, 799–810.

Myers, J. P. (1980). Territoriality and flocking by buff-breasted sandpipers: variations in non-breeding dispersion. *Condor*, **82**, 241–50.

Myers, J. P., Connors, P. G. & Pitelka, F. A. (1979a). Territoriality in non-breeding shorebirds. *Studies in Avian Biology*, **2**, 231–46.
  (1979b). Territory size in wintering sanderlings: the effects of prey abundance and intruder density. *Auk*, **96**, 551–61.
  (1981). Optimal territory size and the sanderling: compromises in a variable environment. In *Foraging Behavior*, ed. A. C. Kamil & T. D. Sargent, pp. 135–58. New York: Garland STPM Press.
Neill, S. R. S. & Cullen, J. M. (1974). Experiments on whether schooling by their prey affects the hunting behavior of cephalopod and fish predators. *Journal of Zoology, London*, **172**, 549–69.
Newman, M. A. (1956). Social behavior and interspecific competition in two trout species. *Physiological Zoology*, **29**, 64–81.
Nice, M. M. (1937). Studies in the life history of the song sparrow. I. *Transactions of the Linneanan Society of New York*, **4**, 1–247.
Nisbet, I. C. T. (1983). Territorial feeding by common terns. *Colonial Waterbirds*, **6**, 64–70.
Nishida, T. (1987). Local traditions and cultural transmission. In *Primate Societies*, ed. B. B. Smuts, D. L. Cheney, R. M. Seyfarth, R. W. Wrangham & T. T. Struhsaker, pp. 462–74. Chicago: University of Chicago Press.
Noirot, E. (1972). The onset of maternal behavior in rats, hamsters, and mice: a selective review. *Advances in the Study of Behavior*, **4**, 107–45.
Nolan, V., Jr. (1963). An analysis of the sexual nexus in the prairie warbler. *Proceedings of the XIII International Ornithological Congress*, 329–37.
Norris, R. A. (1958). Comparative biosystematics and life history of the nuthatches *Sitta pygmaea* and *sitta pusilla*. *University of California Publications in Zoology*, **56**, 119–300.
Norton, M. E., Arcese, M. E., Ewald, P. W. (1982). Effect of intrusion pressure on territory size in black-chinned hummingbirds (*Archilochus alexandri*). *Auk*, **99**, 761–4.
Noske, R. A. (1980). Cooperative breeding by treecreepers. *Emu*, **80**, 35–6.
Nyholm, N. E. I. (1984). Polygyny in the pied flycatcher *Ficedula hypoleuca* at Ammarnas, Swedish Lapland. *Annals Zoologica Fennici*, **21**, 229–32.
O'Brien, S. J., Wildt, D. E., Goldman, D., Merril, D. R. & Bush, M. (1983). The cheetah is depauperate in genetic variation. *Science*, **221**, 459–62.
Ogden, J. C. (1977). Preliminary report on a study of Florida bay ospreys. *National Park Service Transactions and Proceedings*, **2**, 143–51.
Ogden, J. C. & Buckman, N. S. (1973). Movements, foraging groups, and diurnal migrations of the striped parrotfish *Scarus croicensis* Block (Scaridae). *Ecology*, **54**, 589–96.
Orians, G. H. (1961). The ecology of blackbird (*Agelaius*) Social systems. *Ecological Monographs*, **31**, 285–312.
  (1969). On the evolution of mating systems in birds and mammals. *American Naturalist*, **103**, 589–603.
Oring, L. W. (1982). Avian mating systems. *Avian Biology*, **6**, 1–92.
Oring, L. W. & Knudson, M. L. (1972). Monogamy and polyandry in the spotted sandpiper. *Living Bird*, **11**, 59–73.
Oring, L. W. & Lank, D. B. (1986). Polyandry in spotted sandpipers: the impact

of environment and experience. In *Ecological Aspects of Social Evolution*, ed. D. I. Rubenstein & R. W. Wrangham, pp. 21–42. Princeton, NJ: Princeton University Press.

Osborne, D. R. & Bourne, G. R. (1977). Breeding behavior and food habits of the wattled jacana. *Condor*, **79**, 98–105.

Ostfeld, R. S. (1986). Territoriality and mating system of California voles. *Journal of Animal Ecology*, **55**, 691–706.

Owens, D. D. & Owens, M. J. (1979a). Communal denning and clan associations in brown hyenas. (*Hyaena brunnea*, Thunberg) of the central Kalahari Desert. *African Journal of Ecology*, **17**, 35–44.

(1979b). Notes of social organization and behavior in brown hyenas (*Hyaena brunnea*). *Journal of Mammalogy*, **60**, 405–8.

(1984a). Helping behaviour in brown hyenas, *Nature*, **308**, 843–5.

Owens, M. J. & Owens, D. D. (1978). Feeding ecology and its influence on social organization in brown hyenas (*Hyaena brunnea*, Thunberg) of the central Kalahari Desert. *East African Wildlife Journal*, **16**, 113–35.

(1984b). *Cry of the Kalahari*. Boston: Houghton Mifflin.

Owings, D. H. & Coss, R. G. (1977). Snake mobbing by California ground squirrels: adaptive variation and ontogeny. *Behaviour*, **62**, 50–69.

Packer, C. (1986). The ecology of sociality in felids. In *Ecological Aspects of Social Evolution*, ed. D. I. Rubenstein & R. W. Wrangham, pp. 429–52. Princeton, NJ: Princeton University Press.

Page, G. & Whiteacre, D. F. (1975). Raptor predation on wintering shorebirds. *Condor*, **77**, 73–83.

Parmelee, D. F. & Payne, R. B. (1973). On multiple broods and the breeding strategies of Arctic sanderlings. *Ibis*, **115**, 218–26.

Parry, V. (1973). The auxilliary social system and its effect on territory and breeding in kookaburras. *Emu*, **73**, 81–100.

Patterson, I. J. (1965). Timing and spacing of broods in the black-headed gull (*Larus ridibundus*). *Ibis*, **107**, 433–59.

Payne, R. B., Payne, L. L. & Rowley, I. (1984). Splendid wren *Malurus splendens* response to cuckoos: an experimental test of social organization in a communal bird. *Behaviour*, **94**, 108–27.

(1988). Kinship and nest defence in cooperative birds: splendid fairy-wrens, *Malurus splendens*. *Animal Behaviour*, **36**, 939–41.

Peterson, R. O. (1979). The wolves of Isle Royale-new developments. In *The Behavior and Ecology of Wolves*, ed. E. Klinghammer, pp. 3–18. New York: Garland STPM Press.

Petit, K. E., Dixon, M. D. & Holmes, R. T. (1988). A case of polygyny in the black-throated blue warbler. *Wilson Bulletin*, **100**, 132–4.

Petrie, M. (1986). Reproductive strategies of male and female moorhens (*Gallinula chloropus*). In *Ecological Aspects of Social Evolution*, ed. D. I. Rubenstein & R. W. Wrangham, pp. 43–63. Princeton, NJ: Princeton University Press.

Petrinovich, L. & Patterson, T. L. (1978). Polygyny in the white-crowned sparrow (*Zonotrichia leucophrys*). *Condor*, **80**, 99–100.

Picozzi, N. (1983). Two hens, but a single nest: an unusual case of polygyny by hen harriers in Orkney. *British Birds*, **76**, 123–8.

(1984). Breeding biology of polygynous hen harriers *Circus c. cyaneus* in Orkney. *Ornis Scandinavica*, **15**, 1–10.

Pienkowski, M. W. & Green, G. H. (1976). Breeding biology of sanderlings in north-east Greenland. *British Birds*, **69**, 165–77.

Pierotti, R. (1981). Male and female parental roles in the western gull under different environmental conditions. *Auk*, **98**, 532–49.

Pitelka, F. A., Tomich, P. Q. & Treichel, G. W. (1955). Ecological relations of jaegers and owls as lemming predators near Barrow, Alaska. *Ecological Monographs*, **25**, 85–117.

Pleasants, B. Y. (1979). Adaptive significance of the variable dispersion pattern of breeding northern orioles. *Condor*, **81**, 28–34.

Pleszczynska, W. K. (1978). Microgeographic prediction of polygyny in the lark bunting. *Science*, **201**, 935–7.

Pleszczynska, W. K. & Hansell, R. I. C. (1980). Polygyny and decision theory: testing of a model in lark buntings, *Calamospiza melanocorys*. *American Naturalist*, **116**, 821–30.

Plomin, R., DeFries, J. C. & McClearn, G. E. (1980). *Behavioral Genetics*. San Francisco: W. H. Freeman.

Popp, J. W. (1986). Changes in scanning and feeding rates with group size among American goldfinches. *Bird Behaviour*, **6**, 97–8.

Potts, G. R. (1968). Success of eggs of the shag on the Farne Islands, Northumberland, in relation to their content of dieldrin and ppm DDE. *Nature*, **217**, 1282–4.

Poulin, R. & Fitzgerald, G. J. (1989). Shoaling as an anti-ectoparasite mechanism in juvenile sticklebacks (*Gasterosteus* spp.). *Behavioural Ecology and Sociobiology*, **24**, 251–5.

Powell, G. V. N. (1974). Experimental analysis of the social value of flocking by starlings (*Sturnus vulgaris*) in relation to predation and foraging. *Animal Behavior*, **22**, 501–5.

Powell, G. V. N. & Jones, H. L. (1978). An observation of polygyny in the common yellowthroat. *Wilson Bulletin*, **90**, 656–7.

Prescott, D. R. (1986). Polygyny in the willow flycatcher. *Condor*, **88**, 385–6.

Pressley, P. H. (1981). Parental effort and the evolution of nest guarding tactics in the threespine stickleback, *Gasterosteus aculaeatus* L. *Evolution*, **35**, 282–95.

Prevett, J. P. & MacInnes, C. D. (1980). Family and other social groups in snow geese. *Wildlife Monographs*, **71**, 1–46.

Price, F. E. & Bock, C. E. (1973). Polygyny in the dipper. *Condor*, **75**, 457–9.

Price, T. D. & Gibbs, H. L. (1987). Brood division in Darwin's ground finches. *Animal Behavior*, **35**, 299–301.

Prieto, A. A. & Ryan, M. J. (1978). Some observations of the social behavior of the Arizona chuckwalla, *Sauromalus obesus tumidus* (Reptilia. Lacertilia, Iguanidae). *Journal of Herpetology*, **12**, 327–36.

Prior, R. (1968). *The Roe Deer of Cranborne Chase*. Oxford: Oxford University Press.

Pulliam, R., Gilbert, B., Klopfer, P., McDonald, D., McDonald, L. & Millikan, G. (1972). On the evolution of sociality, with particular reference to *Tiaris olivacea*. *Wilson Bulletin*, **84**, 77–89.

Pyke, G. H. (1979). The economics of territory size and time budgets in the golden-winged sunbird. *American Naturalist*, **114**, 131–45.

Quinney, T. E. (1983). Tree swallows cross a polygyny threshold. *Auk*, **100**, 750–4.

Rabenold, K. N. (1984). Cooperative enhancement of reproductive success in tropical wren societies. *Ecology*, **65**, 871–85.

Radabaugh, B. E. (1972). Polygamy in the Kirtland's warbler. *The Jack-Pine Warbler*, **50**, 48–52.

Raitt, R. J., Winterstein, S. R. & Hardy, J. W. (1984). Structure and dynamics of communal groups in the beechey jay. *Wilson Bulletin*, **96**, 206–27.

Ralph, C. P. (1975). Life style of *Coccyzus pumilus*, a tropical cuckoo. *Condor*, **77**, 60–72.

Rau, M. E. (1984). Loss of behavioral dominance in male mice infected with *Trichinella spiralis*. *Primatology*, **88**, 371–3.

Reid, M. L. & Sealy, S. G. (1986). Behavior of a polygynous yearling yellow warbler. *Wilson Bulletin*, **98**, 315–17.

Reyer, H.-U. (1980). Flexible helper structure as an ecological adaptation in the pied kingfisher (*Ceryle rudis rudis* L.). *Behavioural Ecology and Sociobiology*, **6**, 219–27.

(1984). Investment and relatedness: a cost/benefits analysis of breeding and helping in the pied kingfisher (*Ceryle rudis*). *Animal Behaviour*, **32**, 1163–78.

Reynolds, J. D. (1985). Philandering phalaropes. *Natural History*, **94**, 58–65.

(1987). Mating system and nesting biology of the red-necked phalarope *Phalaropus lobatus*: what constrains polyandry? *Ibis*, **129**, 225–42.

Richard, A. (1974). Intra-specific variation in the social organization and ecology of *Propithecus verreauxi*. *Folia Primatologica*, **22**, 178–207.

Richardson, R. A. (1957). Bigamy in swallow. *British Birds*, **49**, 503.

Ridpath, M. G. (1972). The Tasmanian native hen, *Tribonyx mortierii*. II. The individual, the group, and the population. *CSIRO Wildlife Research*, **17**, 53–90.

Rising, J. D. (1987a). Geographic variation in testis size in savannah sparrows (*Passerculus sandwichensis*). *Wilson Bulletin*, **99**, 63–72.

(1987b). Geographic variation of sexual dimorphism in size of savannah sparrows (*Passerculus sandwichensis*): a test of hypotheses. *Evolution*, **41**, 514–24.

Robbel, H. & Child, G. (1975). Notes on territorial behaviour in lechwe. *Mammalia*, **39**, 707–9.

Roberts, S. C. (1987). Group-living and consortships in two populations of the European rabbit (*Oryctolagus cuniculus*). *Journal of Mammalogy*, **68**, 28–38.

Robertson, D. R., Sweatman, H. P. A., Fletcher, E. A. & Cleland, M. G. (1976). Schooling as a mechanism for circumventing the territoriality of competitors. *Ecology*, **57**, 1208–20.

Roell, A. (1979). Bigamy in jackdaws. *Ardea*, **67**, 123–9.

Rolls, J. C. (1983). Probably bigamy by pochard. *British Birds*, **73**, 232.

Rose, R. J., Holaday, J. & Bernstein, I. (1971). Plasma testosterone, dominance rank and aggressive behaviour in male rhesus monkeys. *Nature*, **231**, 366–8.

Rothstein, S. I., Verner, J. & Stevens, E. (1984). Radio-tracking confirms a unique diurnal pattern of spatial occurrence in the parasitic brown-headed cowbird. *Ecology*, **65**, 77–88.

Rowell, T. E. (1974). The concept of social dominance. *Behavioural Biology*, **11**, 131–54.

Rowley, I. (1965). The life history of the superb blue wren. *Emu*, **64**, 251–97.

Rubenstein, D. I. (1980). The evolution of alternative mating strategies. In *Limits to Action: the Allocation of Individual Behavior*, ed. J. E. R. Statton, pp. 65–100. New York: Academic Press.

(1981a). Behavioural ecology of island feral horses. *Equine Veterinary Journal*, **13**, 27–34.

(1981b). Population density, resource patterning, and territoriality in the Everglades pygmy sunfish. *Animal Behaviour*, **29**, 155–72.

(1986). Ecology and sociality in horses and zebras. In *Ecological Aspects of Social Evolution*, ed. D. I. Rubenstein, & R. W. Wrangham, pp. 282–302. Princeton, NJ: Princeton University Press.

Rubenstein, D. I. & Wrangham, R. W. (Eds.) (1986). *Ecological Aspects of Social Evolution*, Princeton, NJ: Princeton University Press.

Ruhiyat, Y. (1983). Socio-ecological study of *Presbytis aygla* in West Java. *Primates*, **24**, 344–59.

Ryan, M. J. (1980). The reproductive behavior of the bullfrog (*Rana catesbiana*). *Copeia*, 108–14.

Sapolsky, R. M. (1987). Stress, social status and reproductive physiology in free-living baboons. In *Physiology and Reproductive Behavior*, ed. D. Crews, pp. 291–322. Englewood Cliffs, NJ: Prentice-Hall.

Savard, J.-P.L. (1986). Polygyny in Barrow's goldeneye. *Condor*, **88**, 250–2.

Schaller, G. B. (1972). *The Serengeti Lion*. Chicago: University of Chicago Press.

Schamel, D. & Tracy, D. (1977). Polyandry, replacement clutches, and site tenacity in the red phalarope (*Phalaropus fulicarius*). *Bird Banding*, **48**, 314–24.

Schemnitz, S. D., ed. (1980). *Wildlife Management Techniques Manual*. Washington, D.C.: The Wildlife Society.

Schuster, R. H. (1976). Lekking behavior in Kafue lechwe. *Science*, **192**, 1240–2.

Scott, M. E. (1988). The impact of infection and disease on animal populations: implications for conservation biology. *Conservation Biology*, **2**, 40–56.

Seghers, B. H. (1974). Schooling behavior in the guppy (*Poecilia reticulata*): an evolutionary response to predation. *Evolution*, **28**, 486–9.

(1981). Facultative schooling behavior in the spottail shiner (*Notropis hudsonius*): possible costs and benefits. *Environmental Biology of Fish*, **6**, 21–4.

Selander, R. K. (1964). Speciation in wrens of the genus *Camphylorhynchus*. *University of California Publications in Zoology*, **74**, 1–224.

Shelley, L. O. (1935). Notes on the 1934 tree swallow breeding-season. *Bird Banding*, **6**, 33–5.

Shugart, G. W. (1980). Frequency and distribution of polygyny in Great Lakes herring gulls in 1978. *Condor*, **82**, 426–9.

Shugart, G. W. & Southern, W. E. (1977). Close nesting, a result of polygyny in herring gulls. *Bird Banding*, **48**, 276–7.

Siegfried, W. R. (1978). Social behavior of the African comb duck. *Living Bird*, **17**, 85–104.

Simmons, K. E. L. (1970). Ecological determinants of breeding adaptations and social behaviour in two fish-eating birds. In *Social Behaviour in Birds and Mammals*, ed. J. H. Crook, pp. 37–77. London: Academic Press.

(1974). Adaptations in the reproductive biology of the great crested grebe. *British Birds*, **67**, 413–37.

Simmons, R. E. (1988a). Food and the deceptive acquisition of mates by polygynous male harriers. *Behavioral Ecology and Sociobiology*, **23**, 83–92.

(1988b). Honest advertising, sexual selection, courtship displays, and body condition of polygynous male harriers. *Auk*, **105**, 303–7.

Simmons, R., Barnard, P., MacWhirter, B. & Hansen, G. L. (1986). The influence of microtines on polygyny, productivity, age and provisioning of breeding northern harriers: a 5-year study. *Canadian Journal of Zoology*, **64**, 2447–56.

Simmons, R., Barnard, P. & Smith, P. C. (1987). Reproductive behaviour of *Circus cyaneus* in North America and Europe: a comparison. *Ornis Scandinavica*, **18**, 33–41.

Skinner, B. F. (1938). *The Behavior of Organisms: an Experimental Analysis*. New York: D. Appleton Century.

Skinner, J. D. (1976). Ecology of the brown hyaena *Hyaena brunnea* in the Transvaal with a distribution map for southern Africa. *South African Journal of Science*, **72**, 262–9.

Smith, A. J. M. (1975). Studies of breeding Sandwich terns. *British Birds*, **68**, 142–56.

Smith, A. T. & Ivins, B. L. (1984). Spatial relationships and social organization in adult pikas: a facultatively monogamous mammal. *Zeitschrift für Tierpsychologie*, **66**, 289–308.

Smith, C. C. (1968). The adaptive nature of social organization in the genus of three squirrels *Tamiasciurus*. *Ecological Monographs*, **38**, 31–63.

(1977). Feeding behaviour and social organization in howling monkeys. In *Primate Ecology*, ed. T. H. Clutton-Brock, pp. 97–126. New York: Academic Press.

Smith, D. M. (1977). *The Social Organization of Rio Grande Turkeys in a Declining Population*. Ph.D. Dissertation, Utah State University.

Smith, J. N. M., Yom-Tov, Y. & Moses, R. (1982). Polygyny, male parental care, and sex ratio in song sparrows: an experimental study. *Auk*, **99**, 555–64.

Smith, S. M. (1967). A case of polygamy in the black-capped chickadee. *Auk*, **84**, 274.

Snow, D. W. (1956). Territory in the blackbird *Turdus merula*. *Ibis*, **98**, 438–47.

Soikkeli, M. (1967). Breeding cycle and population dynamics in the dunlin (*Calidris alpina*). *Annals Zoologica Fennica*, **4**, 158–98.

Sonerud, G. A., Nybo, J. O., Fjeld, P. E. & Knoff, C. (1987). A case of bigyny in the hawk owl *Surnia ulula*: spacing of nests and allocation of male feeding effort. *Ornis Fennica*, **64**, 144–8.

Soule, M. E. (Ed.) (1986). *Conservation Biology: The Science of Scarcity and Diversity.* Sunderland, MA: Sinauer Associates, Inc.

Southern, W. E. (1959). Foster-feeding and polygamy in the purple martin. *Wilson Bulletin*, **71**, 96.

Southwell, C. J. (1984). Variability in grouping in the eastern grey kangaroo, *Macropus giganteus*. I. Group density and group size. *Australian Wildlife Research*, **11**, 423–35.

Srikosamatara, S. & Brockelman, W. Y. (1987). Polygyny in a group of pileated gibbons via a familial route. *International Journal of Primatology*, **8**, 389–93.

Stacey, P. B. (1979a). Habitat saturation and communal breeding in the acorn woodpecker. *Animal Behavior*, **27**, 1153–66.

(1979b). Kinship, promiscuity, and communal breeding in the acorn woodpecker. *Behavioural Ecology in Sociobiology*, **6**, 53–66.

Stacey, P. B. & Bock, C. E. (1978). Social plasticity in the acorn woodpecker. *Science*, **202**, 1298–300.

Stacey, P. B. & Koenig, W. D. (1984). Cooperative breeding in the acorn woodpecker. *Scientific American*, **251**, 114–21.

Stacey, P. B. & Ligon, J. D. (1987). Territory quality and dispersal options in the acorn woodpecker, and a challenge to the habitat-saturation model of cooperative breeding. *American Naturalist*, **130**, 654–76.

Stamps, J. A. (1973). Displays and social organization in female *Anolis aeneus*. *Copeia*, 264–72.

Stamps, J. A. (1986). Conspecifics as cues to territory quality: a preference of juvenile lizards (*Anolis aeneus*) for previously used territories. *American Naturalist*, **129**, 629–42.

Steinbacher, G. (1953). Zür biologie der amsel (*Turdus merula* L.). *Biological Abh.*, **5**.

Stobo, W. T. & McLaren, I. A. (1975). *The Ipswich Sparrow.* Halifax: Nova Scotian Institute of Science.

Stoner, D. (1939). Bird study through banding. *Scientific Monthly*, **49**, 132–8.

Storey, A. E. & Snow, D. T. (1987). Male identity and enclosure size affect paternal attendance of meadow voles, *Microtus pennsylvanicus*. *Animal Behavior*, **35**, 411–19.

Stouffer, P. C., Romagnano, L. C., Lombardo, M. P., Hoffenberg, A. S. & Power, H. W. (1988). A case of communal nesting in the European starling. *Condor*, **90**, 241–5.

Struhsaker, T. T. & Leland, L. (1979). Socioecology of five sympatric monkey species in the Kibale Forest, Uganda. *Advances in the Study of Behavior*, **9**, 159–228.

Swann, R. L. (1975). Communal roosting of robins in Aberdeenshire. *Bird Study*, **22**, 93–8.

Symons, D. (1979). *The Evolution of Human Sexuality.* Oxford: Oxford University Press.

Symons, P. E. K. (1973). Behavior of young Atlantic salmon (*Salmo salar*) exposed to or force-fed fenitrothion, an organophosphate insecticide. *Journal of Fisheries Research Board of Canada*, **30**, 651–5.

(1974). Territorial behavior of juvenile Atlantic salmon reduces predation by brook trout. *Canadian Journal of Zoology*, **52**, 677–9.

Taborsky, M, Hudde, B. & Wirtz, P. (1986). Reproductive behaviour and ecology of *Symphodus* (*Crenilabrus*) *ocellatus*, a European wrasse with four types of male behaviour. *Behaviour*, **102**, 82–118.

Taborsky, M. & Limberger, D. (1981). Helpers in fish. *Behavioural Ecology and Sociobiology*, **8**, 143–5.

Tarbell, A. T. (1983). A yearling helper with a tufted titmouse brood. *Journal of Field Ornithology*, **54**, 89.

Taylor, E. B. (1988). Adaptive variation in rheotactic and agonistic behavior in newly emerged fry of chinook salmon, *Oncorhynchus tshawytscha*, from ocean- and stream-type populations. *Canadian Journal of Fisheries and Aquatic Sciences*, **45**, 237–43.

Teather, K. L. & Robertson, R. J. (1986). Pair bonds and factors influencing the diversity of mating systems in brown-headed cowbirds. *Condor*, **88**, 63–9.

Temrin, H. (1989). Female pairing options in polyterritorial wood warblers *Phylloscopus sibilatrix*: are females deceived? *Animal Behavior*, **37**, 579–86.

Temrin, H. & Jakobsson, S. (1988). Female reproductive success and nest predation in polyterritorial wood warblers (*Phylloscopus sibilatrix*). *Behavioral Ecology and Sociobiology*, **23**, 225–31.

Tener, J. S. (1954). A preliminary study of the musk oxen of Fosheim Island, N. W. T. *Canadian Wildlife Service Wildlife Management Bulletin, First Series*, **9**, 1–34.

(1965). *Musk Oxen in Canada. A Biological and Taxonomic Review*. Ottawa: Department of Northern Affairs and Natural Resources.

Terborgh, J. & Goldizen, A. W. (1985). On the mating system of the cooperatively breeding saddle-backed tamarin (*Saguinus fuscicollis*). *Behavioural Ecology and Sociobiology*, **16**, 293–9.

Terrace, H. S. (1984). Animal cognition. In *Animal Cognition*, ed. H. L. Roitblat, T. G. Bever & H. S. Terrace, pp. 7–28. Hillsdale, NJ: Lawrence Erlbaum Associates.

Townshend, T. J. & Wootton, R. J. (1985). Variation in the mating system of a biparental cichlid fish, *Cichlasoma panamense. Behaviour*, **95**, 181–97.

Trail, P. W. (1980). Ecological correlates of social organization in a communally breeding bird, the acorn woodpecker, *Melanerpes formicivorous. Behavioural Ecology and Sociobiology*, **7**, 83–92.

Trillmich, F. (1978). Feeding territories and breeding success of south polar skuas. *Auk*, **95**, 23–33.

Trivers, R. L. (1972). Parental investment and sexual selection. In *Sexual Selection and the Descent of Man. 1871–1971*, ed. B. Campbell, pp. 136–79. Chicago: Aldine.

Tutin, C. E. G. (1979). Mating patterns and reproductive strategies in a community of wild chimpanzees (*Pan troglodytes schweinfurthii*). *Behavioral Ecology and Sociobiology*, **6**, 29–38.

Tye, A. (1986). Economics of experimentally-induced territorial defence in a gregarious bird, the fieldfare *Turdus pilaris. Ornis Scandinavica*, **17**, 151–64.

Ueda, K. (1984). Successive nest building and polygyny of fan-tailed warblers *Cisticola juncidis. Ibis*, **126**, 221–9.

van Haaften, J. L., Peireira, M. R. & Fonseca, F. P. (1983). A wolf study in Portugal. *XVIth International Congress of Game Biologists*, p. 71.

van Rhijn, J. & Groothuis, T. (1985). Biparental care and the basis for alternative bond-types among gulls, with special reference to black-headed gulls. *Ardea*, **73**, 159–74.

van Schaik, C. P. & van Noordwijk, M. A. (1986). The hidden costs of sociality: intra-group variation in feeding strategies in Sumatran long-tailed macaques (*Macaca fascicularis*). *Behaviour*, **99**, 296–315.

Vaughan, T. A. & Schwartz, S. T. (1980). Behavioural ecology of an insular woodrat. *Journal of Mammalogy*, **61**, 205–18.

Vehrencamp, S. L. (1978). The adaptive significance of communal nesting in groove-billed anis (*Crotophaga sulcirostris*). *Behavioural Ecology and Sociobiology*, **4**, 1–33.

Venables, L. S. V. & Lack, D. (1934). Territory in the great crested grebe. *British Birds*, **28**, 191–8.

(1936). Further notes on territory in the great crested grebe. *British Birds*, **30**, 60–9.

Verner, J. (1964). Evolution of polygamy in the long-billed marsh wren. *Evolution*, **18**, 252–61.

Verner, J. & Willson, M. F. (1966). The influence of habitats on mating systems of North American passerine birds. *Ecology*, **47**, 143–7.

Viitala, J. (1977). Social organization in cyclic subarctic populations of the voles *Clethrionomys rufocanus* (Sund.) and *Microtus agrestis* (L.) *Annales Zoologica Fennici*, **14**, 53–93.

(1980). Myyrien sociologiasta kilpisjarvella. *Luonnon Tutkija*, **84**, 31–4.

Virolainen, M. (1984). Breeding biology of the pied flycatcher *Ficedula hypoleuca* in relation to population density. *Annals Zoologica Fennici*, **21**, 187–97.

vom Saal, F. S. & Bronson, F. H. (1980). Sexual characteristics of adult female mice are correlated with their blood testosterone levels during prenatal development. *Science*, **208**, 597–9.

von Elsner-Schack, I. (1986). Habitat use by mountain goats, *Oreamus americanus*, on the Eastern Slopes region of the Rocky Mountains at Mount Hamell, Alberta. *Canadian Field-Naturalist*, **100**, 319–24.

von Haartman, L. (1951). Successive polygamy. *Behaviour*, **3**, 256–74.

von Schantz, T. (1981). Female cooperation, male competition, and dispersal in the red fox (*Vulpes vulpes*). *Oikos*, **37**, 63–8.

(1984). Carnivore social behavior – does it need patches? *Nature*, **307**, 389–90.

Walker, D. G. (1987). Nest-help and possible polygyny by peregrines. *British Birds*, **80**, 113.

Walkinshaw, L. R. (1959). A chipping sparrow nest in which eight eggs were laid and seven young reared. *Auk*, **76**, 101–2.

Walsberg, G. E. (1977). Ecology and energetics of contrasting social systems in *Phainopepla nitens* (Aves: Ptilogonatidae). *University of California Publications in Zoology*, **108**, 1–63.

Walsberg, G. E. (1978). Brood size and the use of time and energy by the phainopepla. *Ecology*, **59**, 147–53.

Walters, J. R. (1982). Parental behavior in lapwings (Charadriidae) and its relationships with clutch sizes and mating systems. *Evolution*, **36**, 1030–40.

Walther, F. R. (1972). Social grouping in Grant's gazelle (*Gazella granti*) in the Serengeti National Park. *Zeitschrift für Tierpsychologie*, **31**, 348–403.

Ward, I. L. & Weisz, J. (1980). Maternal stress alters plasma testosterone in fetal males. *Science*, **207**, 328–9.

Ward, J. A. & Samarakoon, J. I. (1981). Reproductive tactics of the Asian cichlids of the genus *Etroplus* in Sri Lanka. *Environmental Biology of Fishes*, **6**, 95–103.

Warren, H. B. (1974). Aspects of the behaviour of the impala male, *Aepyceros melampus* during the rut. *Arnoldia*, **6**, 1–9.

Warriner, J. S., Warriner, J. C., Page, G. W. & Stenzel, L. E. (1986). Mating system and reproductive success of a small population of polygamous snowy plovers. *Wilson Bulletin*, **98**, 15–37.

Watanabe, K. (1981). Variations in group composition and population density of the two sympatric Mentawaian leaf-monkeys. *Primates*, **22**, 145–60.

Watson, A. (1957). The behaviour, breeding, and food-ecology of the snowy owl *Nyctea scandiaca*. *Ibis*, **99**, 419–62.

Watts, C. R. & Stokes, A. W. (1971). The social order of turkeys. *Scientific American*, **224**, 112–18.

Weatherhead, P. J. (1979a). Do savannah sparrows commit the Concorde Fallacy? *Behavioural Ecology and Sociobiology*, **5**, 373–81.

   (1979b). Ecological correlates of monogamy in tundra-breeding savannah sparrows. *Auk*, **96**, 391–401.

Welsh, D. A. (1975). Savannah sparrow breeding and territoriality on a Nova Scotia dune beach. *Auk*, **92**, 235–51.

West-Eberhard, M. J. (1989). Phenotypic plasticity and the origins of diversity. *Annual Review of Ecology and Systematics*, **20**, 249–78.

Westneat, D. F. (1987a). Extra-pair copulations in a predominantly monogamous bird: genetic evidence. *Animal Behavior*, **35**, 877–86.

   (1987b). Extra-pair copulations in a predominantly monogamous bird: observations of behaviour. *Animal Behavior*, **35**, 865–76.

   (1988a). Male parental care and extrapair copulations in the indigo bunting. *Auk*, **105**, 149–60.

   (1988b). The relationships among polygyny, male parental care, and female breeding success in the indigo bunting. *Auk*, **105**, 372–4.

Wiklund, C. G. (1982). Fieldfare (*Turdus pilaris*) breeding success in relation to colony size, nest position and association with merlins (*Falco columbarius*). *Behavioural Ecology and Sociobiology*, **11**, 165–72.

Wiley, R. H. & Wiley, M. S. (1980a). Territorial behavior of a blackbird: mechanisms of site-dependent dominance. *Behaviour*, **73**, 130–54.

   (1980b). Spacing and timing in the nesting ecology of a tropical blackbird: comparison of populations in different environments. *Ecological Monographs*, **50**, 153–78.

Williams, G. C. (1964). Measurement of consociation among fishes and comments on the evolution of schooling. *Papers of the Museum of Michigan State University, Biology Series*, **2**, 351–83.

(1966). *Adaptation and Natural Selection*. Princeton, NJ: Princeton University Press.

Willson, M. F. (1966). Polygamy among swamp sparrows. *Auk*, **83**, 666.

Wilson, E. O. (1975). *Sociobiology: The New Synthesis*. Cambridge, MA: Belknap Press.

Wilson, J. (1967). Trigamy in lapwing. *British Birds*, **60**, 217.

Wingfield, J. C. (1984). Androgens and mating systems: testosterone-induced polygyny in normally monogamous birds. *Auk*, **101**, 665–71.

Wingfield, J. C., Ball, G. F., Dufty, A. M., Jr., Hegner, R. E. & Ramenofsky, M. (1987). Testosterone and aggression in birds. *American Scientist*, **75**, 602–8.

Wittenberger, J. F. (1981). *Animal Social Behavior*. Boston: Duxbury Press.

Wobus, U. (1964). Der rothalstaucher (*Podiceps griseigena* Boddaert). *A. Ziemsen*. Lutherstadt: Wittenberg.

Wolf, L. L. (1978). Aggressive social organization in nectarivorous birds. *American Zoologist*, **18**, 765–78.

Wolff, J. O. & Lidicker, W. Z., Jr. (1981). Communal winter nesting and food sharing in taiga voles. *Behavioural Ecology and Sociobiology*, **9**, 237–40.

Wolff, R. J. (1985). Mating behaviour and female choice: their relation to social structure in wild caught house mice (*Mus musculus*) housed in a semi-natural environment. *Journal of Zoology, London*, **207**, 43–51.

Woodward, S. L. (1979). The social system of feral asses (*Equus asinus*). *Zeitschrift für Tierpsychologie*, **49**, 304–16.

Woolfenden, G. E. (1976). A case of bigamy in the Florida scrub jay. *Auk*, **93**, 443–50.

Woolfenden, G. E. & Fitzpatrick, J. W. (1984). *The Florida Scrub Jay: Demography of a Cooperative-Breeding Bird*. Princeton, NJ: Princeton University Press.

(1986). Sexual asymmetries in the life history of the Florida scrub jay. In *Ecological Aspects of Social Evolution*, ed. D. I. Rubenstein & T. W. Wrangham, pp. 87–107. Princeton, NJ: Princeton University Press.

Wootton, J. T., Bollinger, E. K. & Hibbard, C. J. (1986). Mating systems in homogeneous habitats: the effects of female uncertainty, knowledge costs, and random settlement. *American Naturalist*, **128**, 499–512.

Wrangham, R. W. (1983). Social relationships in comparative perspective. In *Primate Social Relationships*, ed. R. A. Hinde, pp. 255–62. Oxford: Blackwell Scientific Publications.

(1986). Ecology and social relationships in two species of chimpanzee. In *Ecological Aspects of Social Evolution*, ed. D.I. Rubenstein & R. W. Wrangham, pp. 352–78. Princeton, NJ: Princeton University Press.

Wynne-Edwards, V. C. (1962). *Animal Dispersion in Relation to Social Behaviour*. Edinburgh: Oliver and Boyd, Ltd.

Ylonen, J. & Viitala, J. (1987). Social organization and habitat use of introduced populations of the vole *Clethrionomys rufocanus* (Sund) in central Finland. *Zeitschrift für Saugetierkunde*, **52**, 354–63.

Yokel, D. A. (1986). Monogamy and brood parasitism: an unlikely pair. *Animal Behavior*, **34**, 1348–58.

228   *References*

Yosef, R. & Pinshow, B. (1988). Polygyny in the northern shrike (*Lanius excubitor*) in Israel. *Auk*, **105**, 581–2.

Zabel, C. J. & Taggart, S. J. (1989). Shift in red fox, *Vulpes vulpes*, mating system associated with El Nino in the Bering Sea. *Animal Behavior*, **38**, 830–8.

Zack, S. (1986). Behaviour and breeding biology of the cooperatively breeding grey-backed fiscal shrike *Lanius excubitorius* in Kenya. *Ibis*, **128**, 214–33.

Zahavi, A. (1971). The social behaviour of the white wagtail *Motacilla alba alba* wintering in Israel. *Ibis*, **113**, 203–11.

Zerbek, N. A. & Butler, R. W. (1981). Cooperative breeding of the northwestern crow, *Corvus kaurinus*, in British Columbia, *Ibis*, **123**, 183–9.

Zezulak, D. S. & Schwab, R. G. (1979). A comparison of density, home range and habitat utilization of bobcat populations of Lava Beds and Joshua Tree National Monuments, California. Paper presented at the Bobcat Research Conference, Front Royal, Virginia, October 15–18, 1979.

Zimmerman, J. L. (1966). Polygyny in the dickcissel. *Auk*, **83**, 534–46.

INDEX

adaptation
  assertion of, 3, 6
  perspective assumed, 99
  social system plasticity as an, 151–4
adaptively neutral variation, 2
aggregation
  forced as a determinant of
    predisposition to form groups, 128
  of grizzly bears, 190–1
alternative mating strategies, 15
ani, 54
  groove-billed, 47, 66, 75, 87, 142
    assessment by, 142
    determinants of communal breeding
      in, 75
    response to predator pressure, 87
  smooth-billed, 25
antelope
  pronghorn, 14, 29, 32, 38, 93, 118, 135,
    163, 182, 186, 189, 192, 193
    social system variation in, 14, 38, 186
    mechanism for change in, 118
    managing effect of sport hunting on,
      14, 189, 192
    as test of socioecological hypotheses,
      182
  African, 162–3, 174
anxiety
  possible proximate determinant of
    grouping, 100
  possible source of assessment
    information, 102, 132
ass, feral, 19, 28, 32, 88
assessment
  availabilty of variables for, 81, 86
  combined with change, 135–6
  costs of, 156–9
  mechanisms breeding birds may use, 53
  mechanisms needed, 9
  potential relationship to developmental
    stages, 105–6

  proximate mechanisms for, 99
  sampling for, 102
  sources of error in, 158–9
  variables that must be assessed, 101,
    138–9, 141–3
Ayu-fish, 27

babbler, grey-crowned, 69
badger, European, 20, 30
bears, Grizzly, 190–1
beaver, 51, 57
bee-eater, red-throated, 69
behavioral gradients, 3
benefits
  of group life, 21–2
  of helping at the nest, 67
  of social system plasticity, 161–2
bison, American, 190
blackbird, 28, 51
  European, 120
  red-winged, 32, 73
  yellow-hooded, 25, 37
bluebird, Eastern, 49, 57
bobcat, 29, 92
bobolinks, 50, 59, 70, 72
bonobo, 174
breeding season
  length of as a determinant of mating
    system, 90
brood split vs. two parent care, 74
  possible processes for, 143, 146
bullfrog, 26
bufflehead, 46
buntings
  indigo, 43, 50, 72
  lark, 50
burro, *see* ass, feral

caracaras
  predatory strategy of, 37, 87, 161

229

secondary reinforcement (*continued*)
  possible proximate mechanism for
    change from solitary to group, 128,
    130, 132
sensitive period
  as a mechanism producing social system
    change, 116
  as a potential assessment process, 104
  in red foxes, 116
sensitization
  possible proximate cause for two-parent
    care in mice, 123
sex ratios
  as a determinant of effective breeding
    population, 185
  as determinants of mating systems,
    60–1, 168–9, 185
  shag, 45, 53
sheep, mountain, 12
shiner, spottail, 17, 127
shrike
  grey-backed fiscal, 70
  northern, 48
shriketit, crested, 69
sifaka, 2, 30
skua
  Arctic, 25
  South Polar, 25, 35
social behavior
  as a manageable resource, 190
social enhancement
  as a mechanism for social system
    change, 119–20
social predispositions, 7
  as a constraint on assumption of
    optimality, 178
  biasing the response to predator induced
    anxiety, 127
  modified by population density,
    predator pressure, nutrition,
    139–40
social relationships
  defined, 3
social strategies
  assessment of, 55
social systems
  background, 4
  classification of, 14
  defined, 3
  versatility of, 164–5
social system plasticity
  benefits of, 12, 161–2
  climate and, 164
  costs of, 12, 156–160
  environmental constraints on, 168
  evolution of, 151–69
  prediction of, 162–9
  psychological complexity and, 167–8
  reproductive biology and, 165–6
  species potential for, 163–4

socioecology
  assumptions made in tests of theory,
    175–9
  history of, 4, 170–1
  hypotheses tested by social system
    variation, 170–82
  model for analysis of social plasticity, 5,
    6
  optimal use of intraspecific variation to
    test hypotheses about, 180–3
solitary, *see* group vs. solitary
spacing systems, 16–41
  possible processes for change, 126–138
  see also, colonial, despotism,
    dominance, flock, group, territory,
    school, undefended home range
sparrow
  chipping, 50, 90
  eastern chipping, 66
  house, 18
  Ipswich, 50
  savannah, 50, 181–2
  song, 50
  swamp, 50
  western lark, 50
  white-browed, 70
  white-crowned, 50, 124
squirrels
  ground, 21
  red, 30
starling
  European, 48, 67
  pied, 70
stickleback, 17, 27, 96, 97
stimulus–response (S–R)
  as a mechanism for behavior
    modification, 109–10
  compared to cognition as an assessment
    mechanism, 134–5
stint, Temminck's, 46, 53, 54, 56, 66
stress
  can reduce testosterone levels, 125
  as a proximate cause of predisposition to
    coloniality, 133
sunbirds
  bronzy, 89, 106, 147–9, 164
  golden-winged, 1, 3–4, 8, 12, 31, 38, 89,
    105, 106, 135, 147, 164, 172, 176–7,
    180
    assessment processes in, 135–6
    assumptions made in study of, 176–7
    determinants of territoriality in, 38
    time spent sitting maximized, 176
sunfish
  green, 31
  pumpkinseed, 31
  pygmy, 27, 31, 40
swallows
  bank, 48, 56
  tree, 43, 48